Acupuncture
for
Migraines

Also by Deborah Bleecker

Natural Back Pain Solutions
Acupuncture Points Handbook
Acupuncture Points Quick Guide
Shingles Relief

Acupuncture for Migraines

How Acupuncture Works for Lasting Relief of Migraine Headaches

Deborah Bleecker, LAc, MSOM

Disclaimer

This book contains the opinions and ideas of the author. It is intended to provide helpful and informative material on the subjects addressed. It is sold with the understanding that the author and publisher are not engaged in rendering medical, health, psychological or any other type of advice or services in the book. If the reader needs personal, medical, health, or other assistance or advice, a competent professional should be consulted.

The author and publisher disclaim any responsibility for any liability, loss or risk, either personal or otherwise that occurs as a consequence, directly or indirectly, of the use and application of the contents of this book.

ISBN 978-1-940146-81-2
Draycott Publishing, LLC

Contents

Acupuncture Restores Blood Circulation and Tissue Oxygen Levels

Introduction

According to most sources, over 38 million people in the US have migraines. It is estimated that 13% of Americans have migraines. What is so shocking to me as an acupuncturist is that most people have no idea that acupuncture and Chinese herbs can completely resolve migraines.

For many years I have explained the basics of what causes migraines to my patients, and how acupuncture treats them. The goal of this book is to put this in writing, so many others can understand the process and get the help they need. There is nothing more heartbreaking than to know that so many people are in agony from migraines and they do not know there is an easy solution.

I asked my patients for testimonials for my website. One of them shocked me. I had no idea what was going on in her head when she first came to see me. I had no doubt that I would be able to completely resolve her migraines. She took the chance and believed me when I tried to explain how I could help. The following is her testimonial:

"I began having migraines at the age of 6. In January 2005, I was having migraines at least 20 days per month. There were days I couldn't get out of bed due to blinding pain, dizziness and nausea. I was on preventative medication and 5 different pain medications.

Every time I saw my neurologist, I left his office with a new prescription. My primary care doctor told me I'd never know what was causing the migraines and that I should learn to live with them.

I was getting my affairs in order because I knew I couldn't live the rest of my life in pain.

Then, after reading about various forms of alternative medicine, I decided to give acupuncture a try.

After just one week, I felt better than I had in years. I am off all medication and I haven't missed a day of work since I began acupuncture treatments.

Deborah literally saved my life. Words cannot express how grateful I am.

In addition to the migraines, I had daily pain in my neck and shoulder due to a pinched nerve. That pain has been eliminated too."

Sarah

It still brings tears to my eyes to realize that Sarah was considering killing herself due to migraine headache pain. I completely understand though. When you are in chronic pain, you wonder why you are supposed to be alive. I have been there myself. I had chronic pain and saw numerous doctors, who were completely unable to help me. Their medicine simply did not treat my type of pain.

Sarah's case is not an unusual one. This is how it works. Get the acupuncture and Chinese herbs you need to address the underlying cause of your migraines, and you too can completely recover.

If you have migraines, or know someone who does, please find an acupuncturist and start care immediately. Do not waste another minute.

Acupuncture and Chinese medicine are a complete solution for all types of headaches and migraines. This book explains exactly how acupuncture works to resolve migraine headaches, as well as other types of associated headaches. It also includes acupressure points so you can help yourself as needed. My goal is to make this information very easy to understand, so you take action immediately.

Even if you have suffered from migraines since you were a child, you can get complete relief from migraines. When you get treatment for the root cause of the migraines, they go away.

Genetic Migraines

There is no such thing as genetic migraines. You might have inherited a tendency to get migraines, but it is not a life sentence. They can be treated, regardless of your family history.

Even if dozens of medical doctors have been unable to help you. Even if you have had multiple injections and taken multiple medications. You can still heal. The answer is to treat your health in a holistic way. When you treat the true root causes of migraines, there is no reason for you to continue having them.

Acupuncture has been used for thousands of years to treat most health issues. It is a complete system of medicine. There are herbal formulas that have been used for over 500 years that are still in use today. They are still used today, because they work!

Practical Guide for Patients

This book is written for non-acupuncturists. I have been treating patients over 20 years and I always wanted a book that explained to patients how acupuncture works to treat migraines.

Migraines are curable. There is no reason to suffer. Your local acupuncturist can help you completely recover from migraines. There are many ways to treat migraines with acupuncture. This book includes information you might find in other textbooks, but I have included my own personal experiences in treating migraines.

Please bear in mind that your acupuncturist might use completely different acupuncture points than I do to heal you. There are many types of acupuncture, and many treatment options. Please remember that your licensed acupuncturist has a degree in Chinese medicine. She will be able to use multiple systems and many different points to heal you. There is no "right" way to do acupuncture. We can adapt the points we use to match each patient exactly.

That is one reason some acupuncture studies are not as successful as you would expect. They often use the same points on every patient. That is not how acupuncture is used by acupuncturists. Acupuncture is so effective because it can be adapted to treat each patient individually, as each patient has a different combination of imbalances that are causing her health problem.

It usually takes only one to three months to completely resolve migraines, regardless of how long you have had them.

I know what it is like to be sick and to not have any idea how or if you can actually recover. In 1994 I had a repetitive stress injury and went to numerous doctors with no relief. I knew if I did not give up, I would find an answer to my health problems. I also knew that medical doctors could not help me, because they told me that, and they exhausted everything they could do and nothing worked. My hope is that this book helps you understand the causes of your migraines, possibly for the first time, as well as how you can get lasting relief.

Although there are many types of migraines, the root cause of all of them is the same. I have not listed all the types of migraines, because the way they are treated is the same. The location of the headache and symptoms are treated using traditional Chinese medicine diagnosis methods that apply to pain in any location.

The acupressure points and herbal suggestions in this book are for informational purposes only. They are not to be used if you are pregnant or might get pregnant. Your licensed acupuncturist will be able to guide you on the best acupressure points to use between acupuncture sessions.

Chapter 1

What Causes Migraine Headaches

There are many possible causes of migraine headaches. In Chinese medicine, pain is caused by a lack of blood circulation. When there is a lack of blood flow, this causes a lack of oxygen also, which causes pain. If there is no blockage of circulation, there will be no pain.

The Chinese medicine theory of what causes pain explains the cause of most types of pain on a basic level. When healthy blood flow is restored, the body can heal itself. The body can always heal itself if you give it what it needs.

Tight muscles put pressure on blood vessels and nerves, disrupting healthy blood flow.

A blockage of circulation anywhere on or near the head or shoulders can easily cause headaches. Some common causes include neck pain, shoulder pain and tightness, hormone imbalances, stress, and sinus headaches.

Acupuncture treats migraines very effectively. In my experience, most patients need a couple of months to treat all the causes of their migraines. After all causes of migraines are addressed, the migraines go away and stay away. Many migraine sufferers have had headaches since childhood, so there are a lot of tight muscles in the head, neck and shoulders that need to be relaxed, as well as sinus and hormone issues are often involved.

One patient only needed about a month of treatment to recover from her migraines. She was very healthy other than the migraines and there was only one cause of migraines. There was a blockage on her forehead, exactly where the headaches occurred.

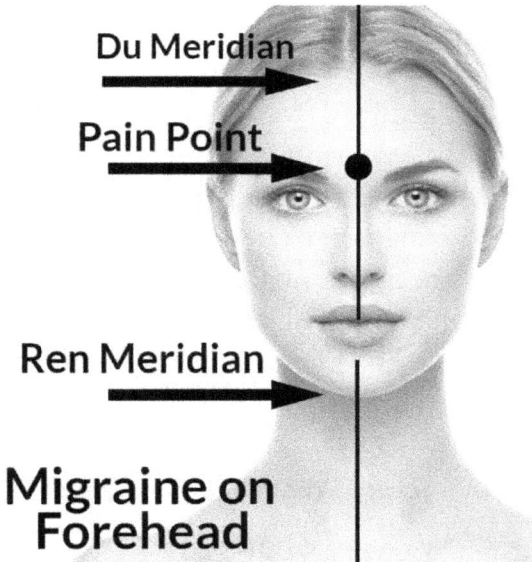

Du Meridian

Pain Point

Ren Meridian

Migraine on Forehead

The image above showed where her headaches hurt. I will explain more on diagnosis and treatment further in the book, but this image shows you how her pain was located on the Du meridian, and I used acupuncture points on her paired meridian, the Ren meridian, on her abdomen, to treat it.

She had been treated by a pain specialist for many years with little relief. Every patient is unique in which meridians are blocked, and the number of other issues causing migraines.

Neck tightness from stress is a common cause of migraines. The neck muscles attach at the base of the skull, and when stress causes neck or shoulder tightness, pressure is put at the base of the skull, blocking healthy blood flow. I see this in the majority of migraine patients. It is easily treated.

Acupuncture Points at Base of Skull

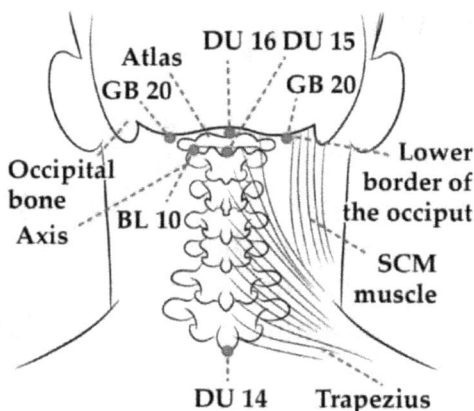

Source: Acupuncture Points Handbook

Throughout this book I will show you images of acupuncture points, and explain how each point treats the cause of migraines. Some of the images are line drawings, which is how acupuncturists learn the points. Some images are photos with dots placed on them. Line drawings make it easy to see the bones and muscle attachments for better point location.

However, I also am including information on how to use acupressure to help yourself. The line drawings are from a point location book I wrote, called *Acupuncture Points Handbook*. This book has over 400 acupuncture points in it.

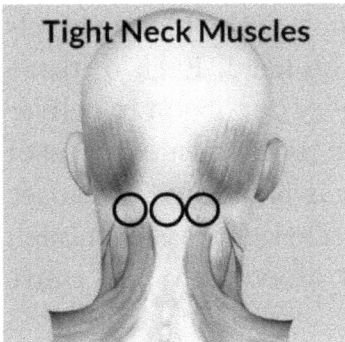

Tight Neck Muscles

This image shows how the muscles from the shoulder go up the neck and attach at the base of the skull. The circles are where many acupuncture points are located.

Acupuncture Is Unbelievable

Most people do not believe that acupuncture can cure migraines. They have suffered so long, and seen so many doctors with little relief. I often have to drag patients kicking and screaming through the process of treatment until they are totally well. I still love treating migraines though, because it is so satisfying to give people their life back after many years of pain.

Another way to understand what causes migraines is to look at the blood vessels and arteries in the head. Each of these blood vessels is very important to deliver oxygenated blood to the tissue. If one of these blood vessels is blocked, it causes pain. Simple muscle tightness is enough to block healthy blood flow and cause pain.

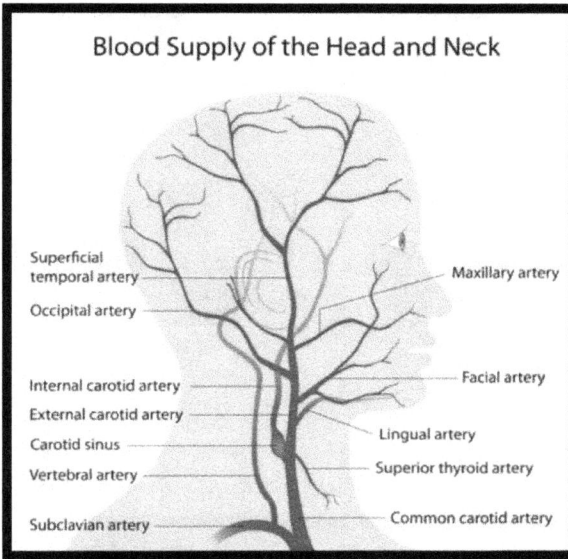

Blood Supply of the Head and Neck

Superficial temporal artery

Occipital artery

Internal carotid artery

External carotid artery

Carotid sinus

Vertebral artery

Subclavian artery

Maxillary artery

Facial artery

Lingual artery

Superior thyroid artery

Common carotid artery

If you notice, this is just the side of the head. There are other branches on other parts of the head that can be blocked. Tight muscles put pressure on these arteries, which causes a lack of healthy blood flow and cellular nutrition to the tissues, which causes pain.

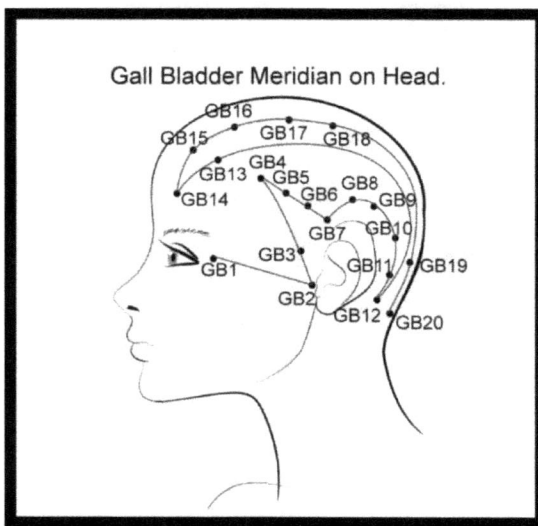

Gall Bladder Meridian on Head.

This image shows how the Gallbladder meridian wraps around the side of the head. The meridian starts by the eye, and there are three lines of the meridian. The meridian also goes through the back of the head. A blockage anywhere on this meridian will cause pain on the head.

Chapter 2

How Acupuncture Treats Pain

Acupuncture treats pain from any cause. Pain is caused by a blockage of circulation. Acupuncture restores circulation in the meridians that are affected, it also breaks down scar tissue, and relaxes tight muscles. When muscles are tight, they put pressure on the nerves, arteries, and blood vessels, which causes pain.

There are actually over 1,000 acupuncture points on the body. TCM, or Traditional Chinese Medicine, includes over 400 commonly used points, but there are other systems of acupuncture such as Ear Acupuncture,

Abdominal Acupuncture, Korean Hand Therapy, Scalp Acupuncture, and many more. Each type of acupuncture will use different points to treat disease.

Distal vs. Local Acupuncture

The acupuncture points used to treat pain can be located on or near the pain, but they can also be located on other areas of the body. There are points on the feet that treat the root cause of migraines. The points work by restoring circulation in the meridian that is affected. Although I usually treat all migraine patients at the base of the skull, as the muscles are often very tight there. I combine these points with other points that treat the root cause of stress, which is the liver in Chinese medicine. This is explained fully in the stress chapter.

The word distal means distant from the affected area. In actuality, other than treating pain exactly on the area of pain, all points are located away from the pain. When acupuncture is done to treat digestive problems, Stomach 36 is used, which is by the knee.

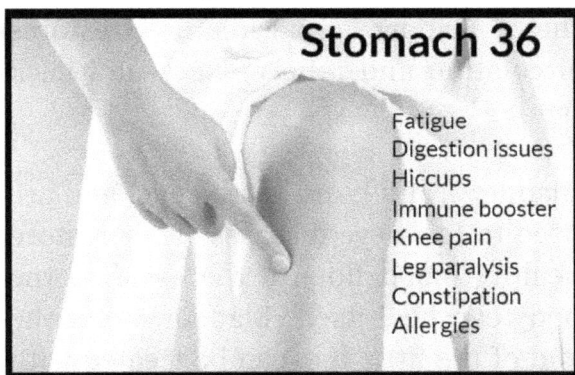

Stomach 36

Fatigue
Digestion issues
Hiccups
Immune booster
Knee pain
Leg paralysis
Constipation
Allergies

If the pain is located on the Gallbladder meridian for example, points on the Gallbladder meridian will restore circulation in the meridians that are affected.

Let's say you have back pain. There are hundreds of points on the body that treat back pain. There are points on the ear, hand, fingers, upper arm, ankles, feet, etc. All of these points restore circulation in that meridian.

The Bladder meridian starts by the eye, and ends at the little toe. There are two

Bladder meridian lines on the back. Treating points on the Bladder meridian, or on a meridian that treats the Bladder meridian, restores circulation and relieves back and neck pain.

Bladder 1 and 2 are by the eye, and are used to treat eye diseases. They restore healthy blood flow to the eyes, so the body can heal itself. Bladder 67, at the end of the little toe, can be treated with moxibustion to turn a breech baby. Bladder 40, which is on the back of the knee, is a very effective point to treat back pain. A blockage anywhere on this meridian will cause pain on the meridian.

Treating on the Opposite Limb

If someone has just had surgery, or a recent accident, it is common to treat them on the opposite side. If there is swelling, doing acupuncture in that area might increase the swelling. It is actually more effective to treat the opposite side of the pain in some cases. It is a judgement call your acupuncturist makes every day.

BL 7
BL 8
BL 9
BL 10

BL 6
BL 5
BL 4
BL 3
BL 2
BL 1

BL 11
BL 12
BL 13
BL 14
BL 15
BL 16
BL 17
BL 18
BL 19
BL 20
BL 21
BL 22
BL 23
BL 24
BL 25
BL 26
BL 31
BL 32
BL 33
BL 34
BL 35
BL 36
BL 37

BL 41
BL 42
BL 43
BL 44
BL 45
BL 46
BL 47
BL 48
BL 49
BL 50
BL 51
BL 52
BL 53
BL 54
BL 30

BL 38
BL 39
BL 40
BL 55
BL 56
BL 57
BL 58
BL 59
BL 60
BL 63
BL 64
BL 65
BL 66
BL 67

BL 61   BL 62

Bladder Meridian

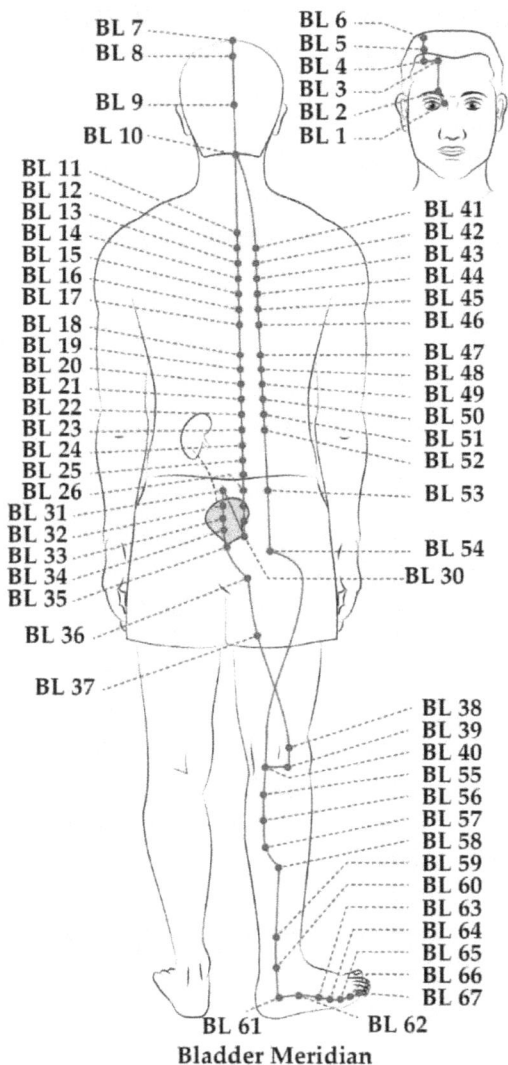

The image above is the Bladder
meridian. It can be used to treat back

pain. There are points on the foot and ankle that activate the Bladder meridian to restore circulation in the back and relieve pain.

The Gallbladder meridian is often affected in migraine patients. This meridian starts by the eye, and travels down to the foot. Most acupuncturists do not put needles in the head for migraine patients, unless someone has a sinus headache. There are points on the face that open the sinuses and relieve sinus pain. Chinese herbal formulas can be used to relieve the inflammation that causes sinus headaches.

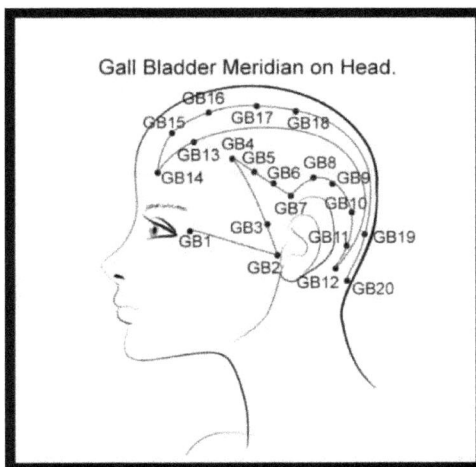

Gall Bladder Meridian on Head.

Inflammation is a cause of pain, but what causes the inflammation? Damage to tissue. When you are injured, your body sends inflammatory chemicals into the area to heal itself. Your body is always trying to heal itself. When there is a lack of blood flow, it is not easy for the body to heal itself. Acupuncture restores healthy blood flow, so the body can heal completely.

Pain is Caused by a Lack of Healthy Blood Flow

Chapter 3

Acupuncture Meridians Explained

The acupuncture meridian system is a network of pathways where energy circulates and connects with the internal organs.

The meridians are used to treat pain, but also the internal organs, which treat internal diseases like fatigue, insomnia, digestive issues, and hormonal imbalances.

Your acupuncturist will determine which meridians are affected. That means that we determine which meridians are blocked. Once we determine which meridians are blocked, we choose points on that meridian, or other points that will treat it.

The needles are tiny, and most people are not bothered by them. After inserting the needles, they are left in for 20-30 minutes, while you relax. Some acupuncturists use TDP or far infrared heat lamps to improve blood flow, which further relaxes the muscles. After 30 minutes, the body has responded to the points that were treated, and the treatment is over.

When a muscle is in spasm, or tight, the acupuncture needle will relax it. Massage or acupressure work the same way. Pressing on a muscle helps to restore blood flow, which relaxes the muscles.

You will often find that odd aches and pains you were not even asking to be treated will resolve when you get acupuncture. When the meridians are treated, that removes obstructions in the meridian and improves blood flow in the entire area.

Most acupuncture points are located on meridians. There are other points, called Extra Points, which are not on regular meridians. When you have pain somewhere, an acupuncturist determines which meridian the pain is located on. After that is determined, she can choose either points on that meridian, or points on other meridians that affect it to treat the pain.

Chapter 4

How Stress Causes Migraines

Stress is a common cause of migraines. The reason stress can cause migraines is that it reduces circulation in the body, it tightens muscles all over, but especially on the head, neck, and shoulders.

You might notice that when you are under stress you are more likely to get headaches. Even if you are not under stress at that very moment, stress builds up in your body. Every stressful event in your life affects your health, and unless it is treated, it will continue to affect your health.

One of my theories about migraines is that people who have migraines from childhood had a stressful childhood. Perhaps they were criticized too much by a family member or other people. This is very common. I have yet to find the person who had a perfect childhood.

All the stress you have ever experienced builds up in your body. If you suppress your feelings, because you were not allowed to express them as a child, the tension gets worse over time. This is a major cause of suicide. The anger that you can have inside from verbal or physical abuse in your childhood is enough to make you want to end it. Chinese medicine has an answer for this. Acupuncture and Chinese herbs can be used to treat the organs that are affected by stress. Over time, your body will become more relaxed and the accumulated stress will not continue to cause health problems.

Bear with me. I know this sounds weird. Each emotion has a corresponding organ that it affects. Too much stress affects your liver. Once your liver is affected, it will continue to be out of balance and will in turn increase your stress levels. It is a vicious cycle.

This is one of the reasons that it takes a while to recover from migraines. The sufferer had to endure the stress of childhood that caused the tight muscles that led to the migraines. The migraines cause stress. Life causes stress. It all builds up and this aspect must be treated for a complete resolution.

If someone has simple muscle spasms, for example causing back pain, that can often be resolved within six visits. But people with migraines have emotional issues, as well as other issues like sinus problems that also need to be resolved. Anything that blocks blood flow to the head or makes the muscles tight can cause pain.

Since the liver is the most common factor in migraines, I will explain it in depth. Bear in mind that most people have some degree of Liver Qi stagnation.

I will only include the most common patterns seen in clinic. There are more patterns that are not very common. If you understand the basics, that is the most important thing.

The following information is sourced from the book *Foundations of Chinese Medicine*, by Giovanni Maciocia. This is the textbook for most acupuncture schools. I will make it as brief and simple as possible.

The Liver (Chinese medicine liver theory) regulates the smooth flow of energy in the body. When it is obstructed or blocked over a long period of time, it can cause depression, frustration, irritability, and emotional tension.

Regular resentment, repressed anger, or depression affect the liver organ (Chinese medicine liver). This causes symptoms such as:

- Chest tightness
- Depression

- Emotional outbursts
- Frequent sighing
- Irritability
- Moodiness
- Muscle tightness
- Nausea
- Premenstrual irritability, stress
- Road rage
- Sensation of something stuck in the throat
- Temper tantrums
- Vomiting

Liver Qi Stagnation (Liver Energy Blockage)

The most common ailment that affects people is Liver Qi Stagnation. Qi is energy or life force. This means that the stress has affected the liver and is now causing obvious symptoms. This also affects the menstrual cycle. It causes menstrual cramps, period irregularity, infertility, and depression. If your liver energy is stagnant, it is impossible to be stress free or relaxed. The good news is that Chinese medicine can diagnose and treat all these things. There are acupuncture points and Chinese herbal medicine formulas that treat this imbalance. This treats the root cause of stress, and many other health issues.

Liver stagnation often causes excess heat in your body. You might find you sweat more than other people, or get a flushed face when you are angry.

Common points to treat this disease are located on the Liver meridian. Liver 3 is a very commonly used acupuncture point. Everyone needs it. It is located in the hollow area between the foot bones. If you place your finger on the area shown in the image, you will feel a slight hollow area.

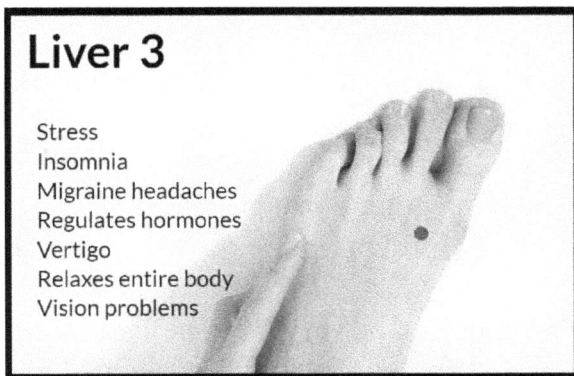

Liver 3

Stress
Insomnia
Migraine headaches
Regulates hormones
Vertigo
Relaxes entire body
Vision problems

Liver Qi stagnation can lead to other types of liver pathologies. All menstrual disorders can be treated with Chinese medicine. They are often due to liver imbalances. Your symptoms tell us how your body is out of balance.

A commonly prescribed herbal formula for this pattern is Jia Wei Xiao Yao San. This formula is amazing to treat stress. It works by regulating the liver energy.

Liver Blood Stasis

A less common type of liver imbalance is liver blood stasis. This is a severe form of liver imbalance that is caused by severe stress over a long period of time. The most common symptoms are:

- Dark clotted blood during the period
- Infertility
- Irregular periods
- Painful periods

The clots can be very large in liver blood stasis. The woman who has liver blood stasis will often feel a sense of relief after passing the clots during her period. I would say this is a fairly uncommon problem, but I wanted to mention it in case it applies to you or someone you know. This is a very treatable menstrual problem. Your acupuncturist can use acupuncture and Chinese herbal medicine to regulate your hormones and resolve this problem.

Liver Fire

This is a common liver imbalance. This can easily cause neck and shoulder pain also. This is a severe type of imbalance. I would say that most people who have road rage probably have Liver Fire. If they would get acupuncture and take herbs, they would calm down and life would be better for everyone. The most common symptoms of Liver Fire are:

- Bitter taste in the mouth
- Dizziness
- Headaches on the temples
- Rage
- Red eyes
- Red face

41

- Severe irritability
- Tinnitus
- Flushed face when irritated or angry

As an acupuncturist, I will look at your tongue, and take your pulse to determine which type of liver imbalance you have. In addition, I like to ask if someone has a flushed face when they get mad. If you get a red or hot face when under stress or mad, your liver is on fire. Chinese medicine can treat it.

You will find that when people in your life have Liver Fire, they tend to make you have Liver Fire. They are irritable and it affects everyone around them.

A commonly used point to treat Liver Fire is Liver 2. The herbal formula for this is Long Dan Xie Gan Tang. This formula should not be taken long term. Patients usually take it less than 30 days, then other imbalances are treated. If you have Liver Fire, I think you will be pleasantly surprised to see how fast you get relief with Chinese herbs. Most people feel a lot calmer in a few days after starting acupuncture and herbs.

As you can see in the image of Liver 2, it is located in the web between the first and second toes.

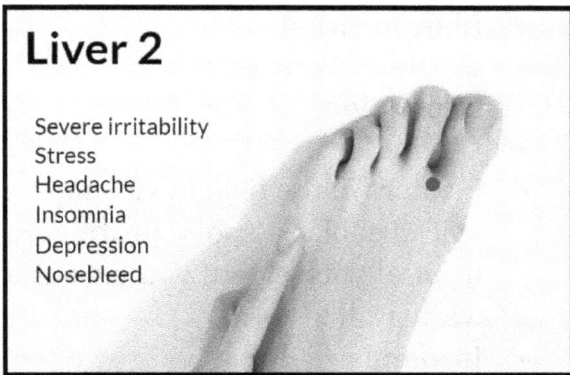

Liver 2

Severe irritability
Stress
Headache
Insomnia
Depression
Nosebleed

Liver Blood Deficiency

This pattern involves not having enough blood in the liver. It sometimes correlates to anemia, but not always. It can be a precursor to anemia. Chinese medicine catches health problems before Western medicine is able to pinpoint what the problem is.

Because women lose blood with their monthly cycle, this is more common in women. Your body has to create more blood every month to replace what is lost during the period. If it cannot do this, it can cause liver imbalances, and other problems. The most common symptoms of liver blood deficiency are:

- Blurred vision
- Brittle nails
- Depression
- Dizziness
- Floaters in the field of vision, you will see black spots floating in front of your eyes if you look at a white wall
- Insomnia
- Muscle cramps
- Muscle pain
- Night vision reduced
- Numbness of the arms or legs
- Pale face
- Pale lips
- Period stops entirely or is irregular
- Ridges in fingernails
- Scanty menstrual blood
- Scanty periods
- Tight muscles

I have had patients who had stopped having a period in their twenties or thirties who were told that they were in early menopause. They were simply liver blood deficient. This is easy to treat with Chinese medicine. If you have a menstrual problem, the first thing you need to do is get acupuncture and take Chinese herbs. This applies also to infertility. Before you want to get pregnant, get acupuncture a couple of months to prepare your body and improve fertility. Acupuncture is amazing for fertility.

In order to restore healthy blood in the liver, several things need to be treated. The liver needs to be treated, but the digestion needs to be treated also. Sometimes weak digestion causes a lack of healthy nutrients in the blood.

Depression

Liver blood deficiency can easily cause depression. Emotional issues have a root cause in an imbalance in the body. You cannot separate the emotions from the health of the body. Chinese medicine excels at treating emotional issues.

To boost energy levels and improve digestion Stomach 36 is a good option. Stomach 36 is one of the most important points on the body, it has many functions.

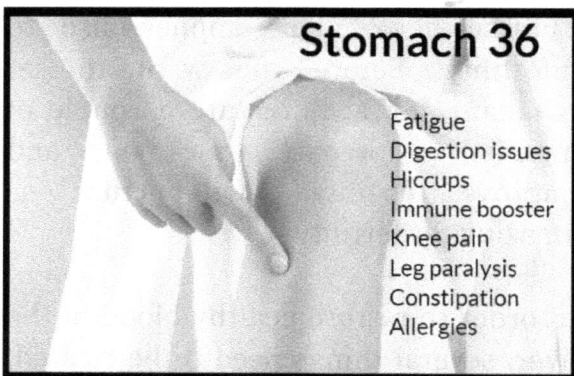

Stomach 36

Fatigue
Digestion issues
Hiccups
Immune booster
Knee pain
Leg paralysis
Constipation
Allergies

Spleen 6 is the premier point to improve blood production and regulate hormones. It also helps rid the body of excess fluid. It also treats emotional issues and infertility.

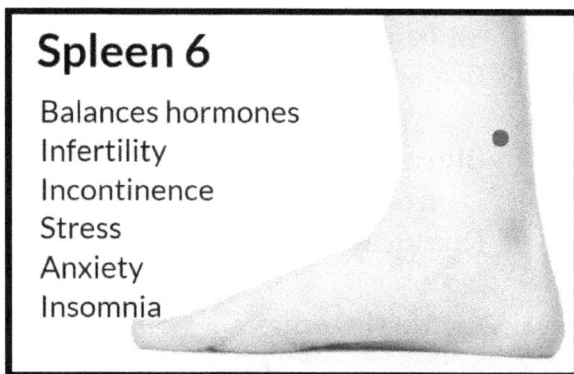

Spleen 6

Balances hormones
Infertility
Incontinence
Stress
Anxiety
Insomnia

Depending on the severity of liver blood deficiency, the herbal formula Jia Wei Xiao Yao San can often resolve the problem. This formula is very commonly used and is sold in stores in China. The long tradition of using Chinese herbs to treat disease means that people often take herbs to help themselves if their problem is not serious.

Liver Yin Deficiency

This is not a common cause of migraines, but it is possible. It often occurs in women over 45, and certainly over 50. The Yin can be described as estrogen. It is much more than estrogen, but that is the easiest way to describe it.

47

The most common symptoms of a Liver Yin Deficiency are:

- Blurred vision
- Depression
- Dizziness
- Dry eyes
- Brittle fingernails
- Floaters in the eyes
- Insomnia
- Muscle cramps
- Muscle weakness
- Night vision impaired
- Scanty menstrual blood, or lack of menstruation
- Very dry hair

Dry eyes are very common in people over 50. There are herbal formulas that treat this. This has nothing to do with migraines, but I wanted you to know.

To restore the yin of the liver Spleen 6 is used, Stomach 36, and Liver 3. In addition, points on the Kidney meridian restore the kidneys, and also the hormones. The kidney points can be used to treat kidney imbalances that cause things like frequent or urgent urination, incontinence, fatigue, excess fluid in the body (edema), and back pain.

Kidney 7 is commonly used to treat urinary disorders like incontinence. Kidney 6 can be used for Kidney yin, as well as hot flashes.

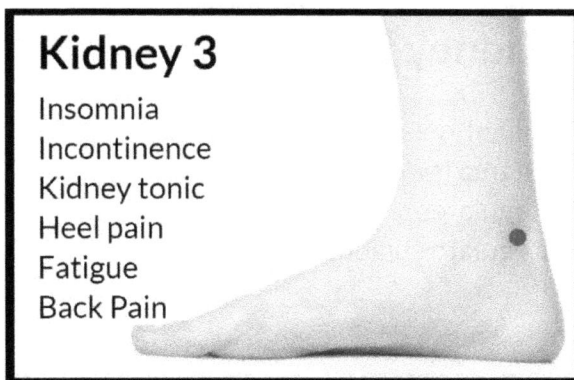

Kidney 3

Insomnia
Incontinence
Kidney tonic
Heel pain
Fatigue
Back Pain

Kidney 6

Hot flashes
Calms mind
Insomnia
Sore throat
Moistens throat

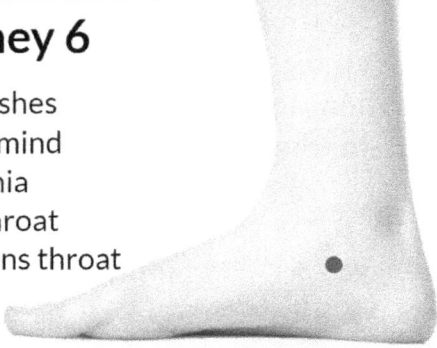

Kidney 7

Incontinence
Edema (swelling)
Regulates sweating
Regulates bladder

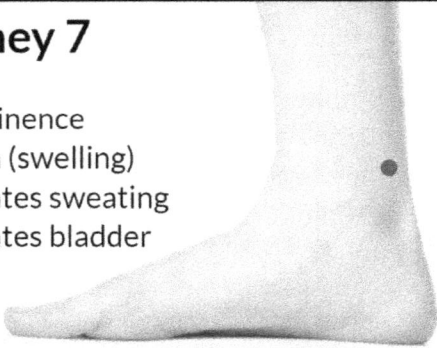

Liver Yang Rising

I know this is a particularly weird title for this disorder. In Chinese medicine, the liver energy can go up to the head, instead of down, as it should. When it does this, it can cause common symptoms such as:

- Angry outbursts
- Blurred vision
- Dizziness
- Dry mouth and throat
- Headache by the eyes, temples, or sides of head
- Insomnia
- Irritability
- Stiff neck
- Tinnitus

This pattern is also often associated with high blood pressure. In Chinese medicine theory, the yin is not strong enough to keep the liver energy from going to the head. I believe the modern correlation with this is that the liver is clogged as you age, and this prevents the liver from processing the chemicals that reduce blood pressure.

Common points to treat this pattern are as previously shown, Spleen 6, Stomach 36, Kidney 3, Kidney 6, and Liver 2. Notice how these points can be used for so many ailments. There is no down side to using extra points for each ailment.

Numerous points will be used, because it is the rare person who only has one organ pattern imbalance.

The liver is the most common cause of migraines, but it is not the only one, and other issues can be addressed at the same time as the migraines are treated. That is how acupuncture works.

If you have insomnia, we treat that at the same time as the migraines. Fatigue, anxiety, depression, digestive problems, everything is treated, so when your treatment time is over and your migraines are gone, your other ailments are also gone. We do not isolate symptoms and treat one thing at a time, because everything works together in your body. If you are not getting enough sleep, it will be hard to heal. If you are anxious, that affects your sleep and your stress also.

Rebellious Liver Qi Invading the Stomach

This is a doozy. This sounds nuts to a non-acupuncturist. When the liver energy is out of balance, it can actually invade other organs energetically. In addition to the common symptoms of liver imbalance, you will have digestive or stomach issues. I have recently heard about abdominal migraines. I have not treated them, but I believe they are associated with this organ pattern.

The common symptoms of this pattern are:
- Acid reflux
- Belching
- Feeling of oppression above the stomach
- Hiccups
- Irritability
- Nausea
- Sighing frequently
- Stomach area distension and pain
- Vomiting

The American Migraine Foundation has the following information on their site:

"Abdominal migraine is a sub-type of migraine seen mainly in children. It consists of episodes of abdominal pain with nausea, vomiting, loss of appetite or pallor. Between episodes, there should be no symptoms. Children with abdominal migraine generally go on to develop migraine headaches later in life. People suspected of having abdominal migraine should be carefully assessed by their doctor for an underlying cause as certain gastrointestinal, urogenital or metabolic conditions may mimic abdominal migraine."

Abdominal Migraines:

- Abdominal pain with nausea
- Loss of appetite
- Vomiting

If I had a patient with the above symptoms, I would balance the liver with Liver 2 and Liver 3. In addition, I would treat digestion with Stomach 36. I would also treat the Ren meridian, which is very strong to regulate the stomach. Ren 12 is shown in the image below. It is located one hand width above the belly button.

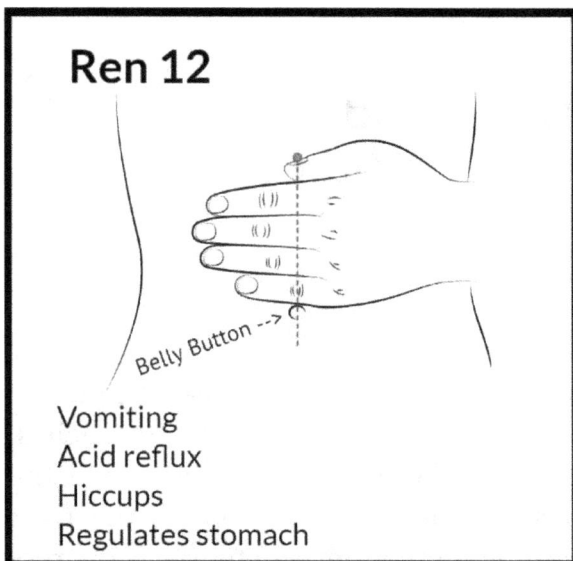

Ren 12

Belly Button -->

Vomiting
Acid reflux
Hiccups
Regulates stomach

As you can see, stress causes many health problems. Everyone could benefit from getting acupuncture and taking Chinese herbs to treat this. Stress is not going to go away on its own, but it can be treated. This is a very important aspect of treating migraines, relieving the stress that often causes the headaches in the first place.

Chapter 5

Neck and Shoulder Pain Migraines

When the shoulder and neck muscles are tight, they can easily cause headaches. Some of the neck muscles attach at the base of the skull. Over time, the tight muscles get tighter and tighter and press on the nerves and blood vessels. This stops blood flow, which causes pain. Once you relax the muscles, the pain goes away.

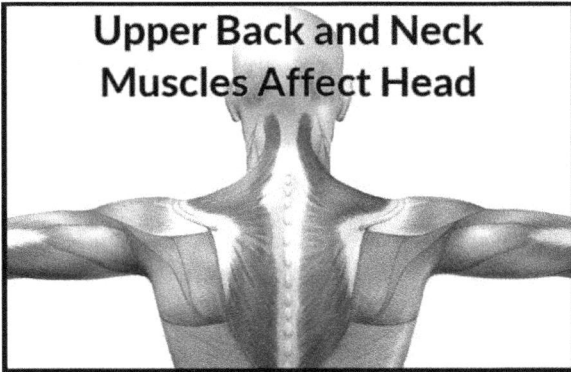

Upper Back and Neck Muscles Affect Head

The image above is of the trapezius muscle. In the second image you can see that the muscle is located on the upper back, neck, and even the front side of the neck. Tension anywhere on this muscle can put pressure on nerves, and blood vessels which can easily cause pain.

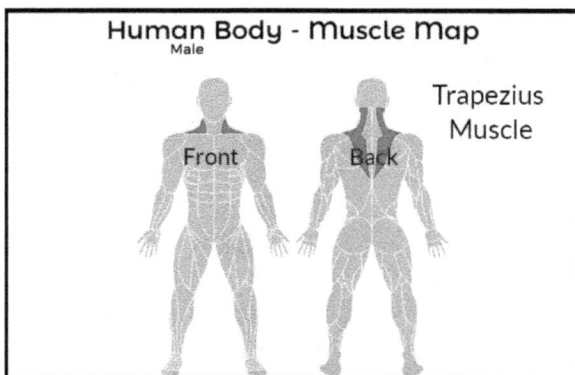

When I treat migraines, I usually treat the neck and shoulders on the second treatment. I want to make sure that if there are any tight muscles in the area they can start to relax. The reason I usually wait until the second treatment is that most patients are uncomfortable being face down for their first acupuncture treatment. Once I do the first treatment on the front of the body, they learn that it is not nearly as bad as they thought it would be, in fact they often barely feel the needles.

There are a lot of muscles in the neck. Any one of these muscles can be tight and cause a blockage anywhere in the neck or shoulders which causes migraines. In addition, when muscles are tight over a long period of time, they are similar to scar tissue. The needles will break down the scar tissue, but it will take time to treat all of it, as scar tissue can be present in numerous locations, all causing blocked circulation.

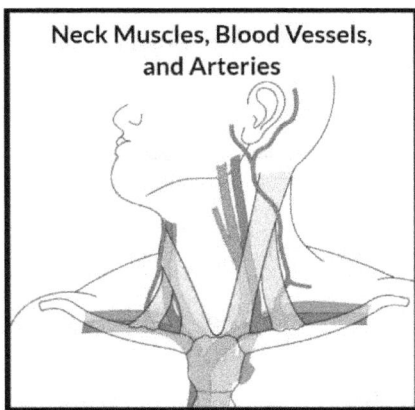

Neck Muscles, Blood Vessels, and Arteries

Chronic inflammation causes scar tissue. Inflammation is your body trying to heal the area. When there is a lack of blood flow, it cannot complete the healing. Acupuncture restores healthy blood flow so the body can heal itself.

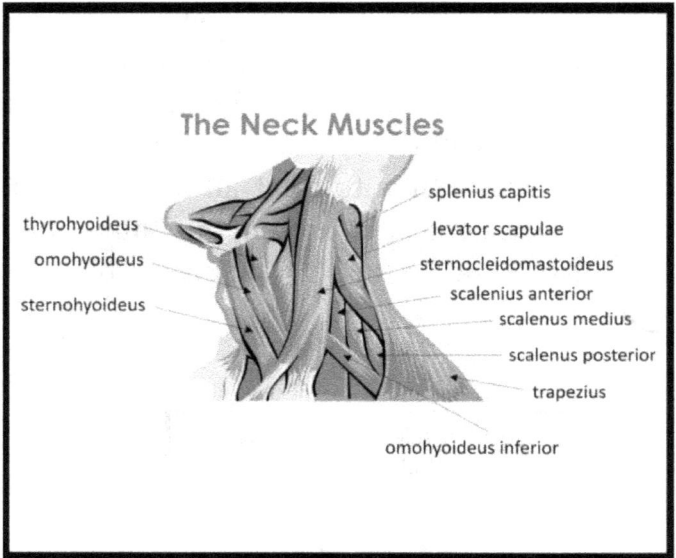

The Neck Muscles

thyrohyoideus
omohyoideus
sternohyoideus

splenius capitis
levator scapulae
sternocleidomastoideus
scalenius anterior
scalenus medius
scalenus posterior
trapezius

omohyoideus inferior

Healing Time

The headaches will get weaker and less frequent over time. Most people have many health issues that affect healing. If you have a job that is stressful, or anything that continues to stress you out, that will slow down healing. Stress causes tight muscles. The way that acupuncture works to treat pain is that you might not feel much on your first treatment. Your body develops pain patterns that it has to break. Many muscles are involved, and they all need to be treated.

After a few acupuncture treatments, you will find that your migraines are not as strong, then they occur less often, and this continues over time, until they are gone completely. If you do not have migraines every day, that is OK. We will treat the underlying cause of the migraines, so they are less likely to come back.

There are several herbal formulas that treat stress. Sometimes it is necessary to address stress with Chinese herbal medicine before the neck muscles can relax.

I had a patient who had neck pain. I treated his neck as I always do, but he got little relief. I finally determined that he was so stressed out, and had been for a long time, that he would not get better until we calmed his body down with strong Chinese herbal formulas. After a couple of weeks of stress herbs, his neck pain went away.

In his case, he had liver fire and his entire body was very tight due to stress. After he took the formula Long Dan Xie Gan Tang, the acupuncture was effective to relieve his neck pain. I had not had this happen before, but this demonstrates how each patient can have different causes for their pain.

There are several ways to treat neck pain. There are points on the hands and feet that treat the neck, there are points on the neck itself, and on the base of the skull, where the muscles attach. I also like to use ear acupuncture to treat the neck.

Ear Acupuncture
The entire body can be treated via the ear. The ear can be mapped using the image of an inverted fetus. That shows where each body part is represented on the ear. I use tiny ionic ear seeds on the area related to the neck. The patient can wear them for a few days and press on them as needed for neck pain. This is a great way to fill in the gaps when a

patient does not get acupuncture every day.

Most patients get acupuncture twice a week. If you are in an emergency situation and your migraines have not been reduced enough, three times a week is a good schedule until you are stabilized. The severity of the migraines usually goes down quickly.

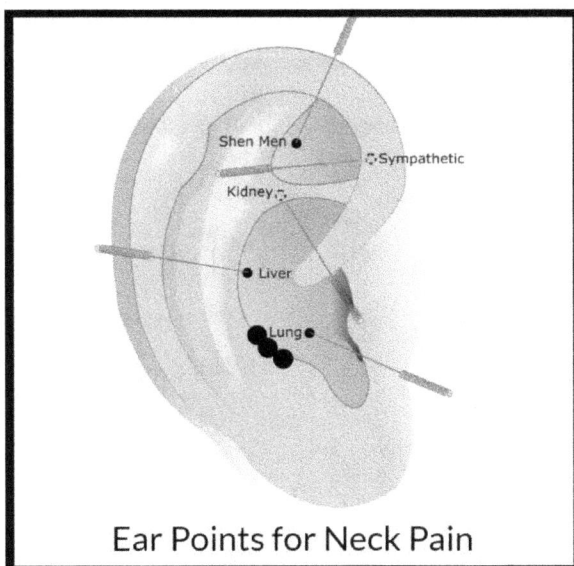

Ear Points for Neck Pain

The Gallbladder meridian starts by the eye and wraps around the head several times, goes down to the base of the skull, then ends at the foot. There are acupuncture points on the foot that treat pain on the Gallbladder meridian. The Gallbladder meridian is commonly involved in migraines.

If you see the path of the meridian, you can see that tight muscles on the neck can put pressure on the Gallbladder meridian, blocking it.

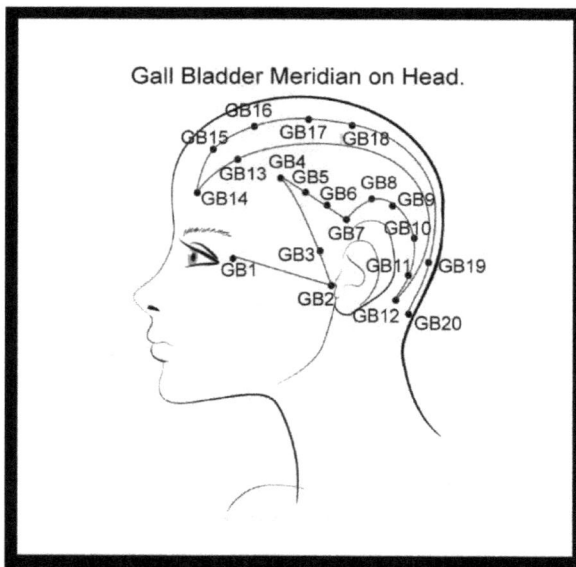

Gall Bladder Meridian on Head.

Stretches for Neck and Shoulder Tightness or Pain

Stretching is very important to relieve tense muscles in the shoulders and neck. It is especially important if you sit at a desk all day. It is easy to tend to slump forward. This causes the muscles to shorten and put pressure on the nerves, which causes pain.

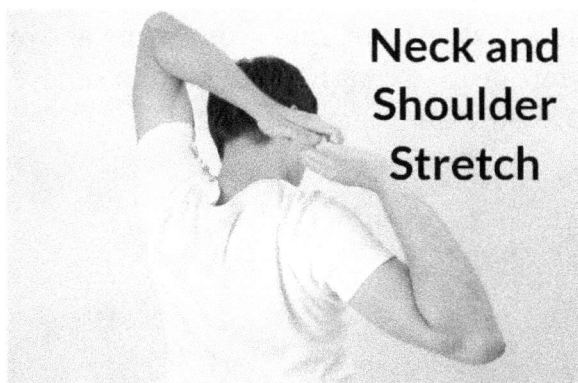

Neck and Shoulder Stretch

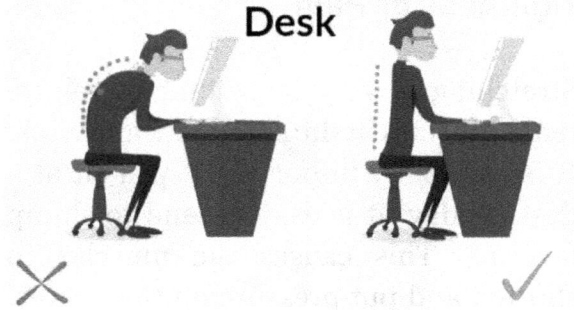

Bad Posture when Sitting at Desk

Stretching can be very simple. If you sit at a desk all day, raise your arms above your head. Even that will help to relieve pressure and relax muscles.

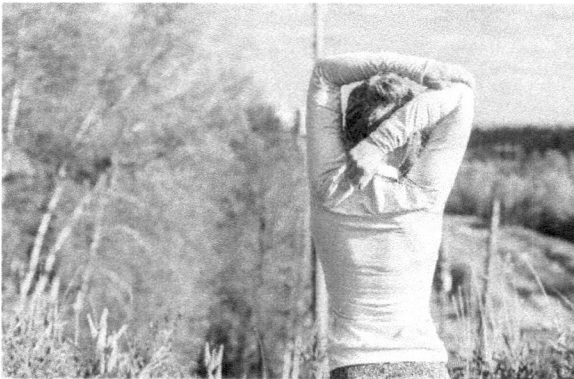

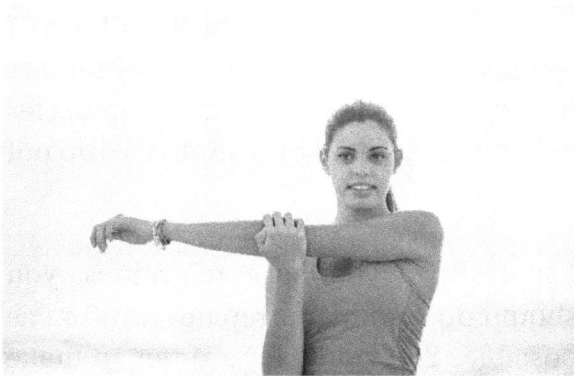

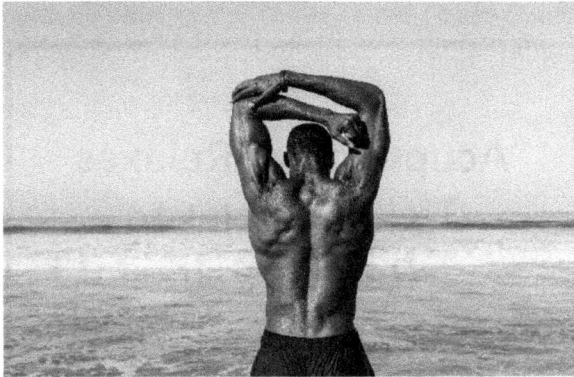

I used to have thoracic outlet syndrome, which is shoulder pain and nerve problems caused by tight muscles in the shoulders. I found that stretching was one of the most important parts of my healing. The image above, of the man at the beach, is the most important stretch I do when typing all day. I hold my arms like that and pull them back as far as I can and hold it 5-10 seconds. We tend to be very still when we sit. Our muscles will just tighten up over time if we do not move them.

Especially if you have migraines, you should do shoulder stretches as often as possible. You could set a timer to make sure you do it at least once an hour.

Acupuncture Relaxes Tight Muscles to Relieve Pain

Neck Pain and Pillows

Sometimes people use pillows that are too high. If the pillow is too high it can put pressure on the neck and irritate the nerves, which can cause headaches. Memory foam pillows often cause problems when the head sinks down into them and it cannot move freely during the night.

Pillows that are too hard can easily cause neck and head pain. I personally like down-like pillows. They do not have to be expensive. The image below shows how a pillow that is too high puts pressure on the neck and back.

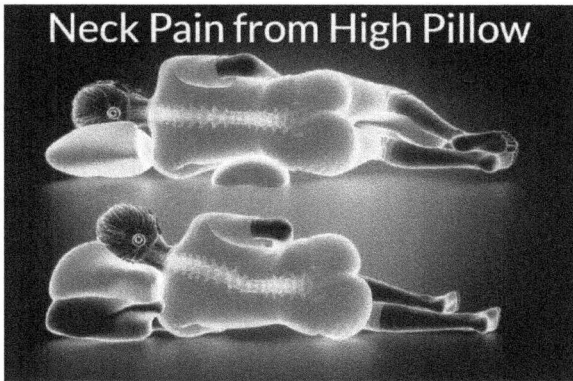

Neck Pain from High Pillow

Car Accidents and Whiplash

People often underestimate how damaging car accidents are. I am a lot more concerned about the personal injuries people have than how their car is.

Don't let anyone discount your pain if you have been in an accident. It causes physical and emotional distress that takes time to heal. When you are jolted around, damage is done to the tendons, ligaments, and discs in the spine. This causes inflammation that can cause headaches.

Please consider getting acupuncture as soon as possible after a car accident. It will relax muscles and restore blood flow to inflamed tissue, so it can heal.

Notice how the head is violently jolted back and forth in whiplash. You will not always feel the pain on the day of the accident. Shock keeps you from feeling pain sometimes, and your body compensates by altering posture, which causes different types of pain later.

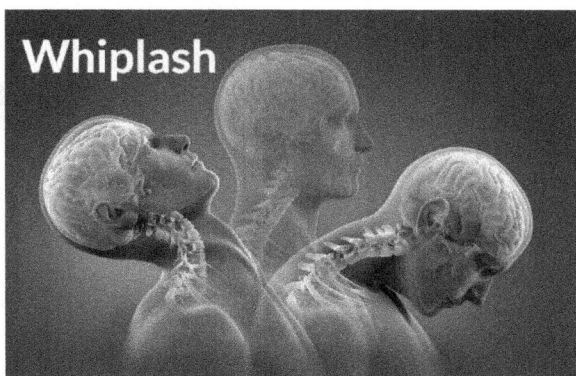
Whiplash

Chapter 6

Sinus Headache Migraines

Sinus headaches can easily cause severe headaches and migraines. The sinuses take up a very large area on the head, and when they are inflamed, they swell up and can put pressure on nerves, which causes pain.

There are acupuncture points that open the sinuses and relieve pain, and there are herbal formulas that treat the underlying inflammation and allergic reaction.

A common cause of sinus problems is eating dairy. Any food allergy can inflame your sinuses, but dairy is the most common. It causes an allergic reaction because it contains sugars and milk proteins that your body cannot easily digest, so it can cause an immune response.

Pain on Your Face

If you have pain anywhere on your face, jaw, or ears, consider it might be caused by sinus problems.

Notice how deep the sinuses go in the image below.

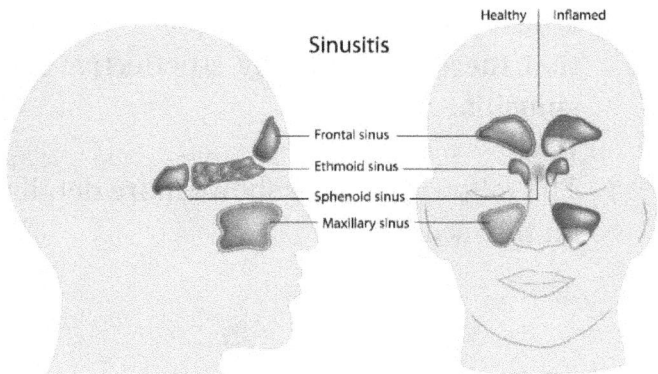

Most images only show the sinuses from the front. It is easy to see how the sinus areas and where it might hurt, but if you see it from the side, you can see how

73

deep they go, and how profoundly they can impact headaches when they are inflamed.

There is no need or benefit to have sinus surgery. From what I understand, they just scrape out the inside of the sinuses. There are so many herbal formulas in Chinese medicine that treat sinus inflammation quickly. Most people do not believe me until I give them a few capsules of the formula. Within 30 minutes to an hour, the sinus pain is gone and they want their own bottle. It is just hard for most people to believe that there is something so effective for sinusitis.

The following image shows more details on the face.

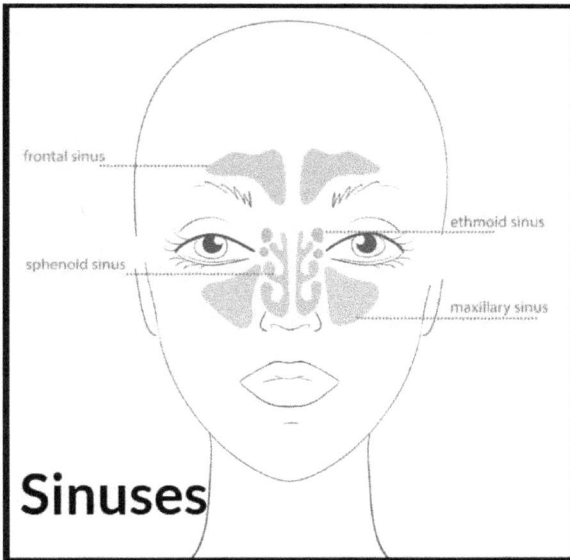

frontal sinus

ethmoid sinus

sphenoid sinus

maxillary sinus

Sinuses

In the acupressure chapter, I will show you how to do acupressure to relieve sinus pain quickly. In a pinch, you can try ginger root to relieve sinus problems and headaches in general. It relieves inflammation. I take two tablets of a ginger extract from Planetary Herbals. If that is not available, I take four to six tablets of the raw herb from Solaray or Nature's Way.

Sinus problems can also be caused by Candida. The fungus or another fungal growth can grow in your sinuses.

North American Herb and Spice makes a sinus spray that can help relieve sinus pain. It is called Sinu Orega. It has oregano and other herbs that clear infection, and they are natural anti-fungals.

Chapter 7

Botox Injections

Botox is increasingly being used to treat migraines. Botox is an extract of Botulinum toxin. Yes, it is a toxin. It basically paralyzes the nerves temporarily. When the nerves are basically paralyzed, that prevents them from tightening the muscles.

Botox has been used for years on the face, to reduce common frown expressions by the eyes. After analyzing people's faces, I have noticed that often their eyes do not look as sparkly and healthy after getting injections. I believe that is because healthy blood flow has been impaired.

ACUPUNCTURE FOR MIGRAINES

Acupuncture can also be used to do acupuncture facelifts, or facial acupuncture. I often use a few extra needles on my patients to relax their faces so the frown lines go away. It is not difficult. You will usually see the results of the relaxed muscles after the first treatment. Each time you get acupuncture it relaxes the muscles more and the face is essentially very relaxed. The eyelids can be lifted by treating the eyes. Wrinkles, like pain, are caused by tight muscles. When the muscles are tightened repeatedly, they eventually stay that way. As we age, the skin starts to sag due to a reduction in collagen, and reduced blood flow. Acupuncture can help this also, by improving blood flow and restoring normal function.

I believe that the most common locations to inject Botox are at the base of the skull. I have already mentioned how tight muscles that attach to the base of the skull are often involved in migraines. Whether the pain originates from there or somewhere else, it often ends up affecting those muscles.

I believe in doing whatever you have to do to get out of pain fast. But acupuncture also helps you get out of pain fast, and it is not toxic. Nothing is injected, and there are no long-term side effects on the nerves.

If a person gets Botox injected, and the nerves are paralyzed for a period of time, it is not known if there are long term side effects. The reason I mention this is that acupuncture theory explains many health issues by treating acupuncture points that restore circulation to the area that is diseased. There are points around the eyes that are used to effectively treat many eye diseases.

If the theory is that restoring healthy blood flow can help the body heal itself, what happens when you block circulation on purpose? Will there be lasting damage? I do not believe we know right now if these Botox injections affect future diseases. I am not claiming that they do, but it is something to consider.   Your body wants healthy blood flow in ALL tissues. That is how you stay healthy. Your body heals itself every day, if you give it what it needs.

Pain is Caused by a Lack of Healthy Blood Flow

If People Tell You That You That Migraines Are Incurable, Ignore Them and Get Acupuncture!

Chapter 8

Chinese Herbal Medicine for Migraines

Chinese herbs are 50% of Chinese medicine. If you do not take herbs from a qualified herbalist, you are cheating yourself.

If you take herbs as prescribed, you can get better much faster, at lower overall cost. It is not required, but it is a huge benefit if you can take Chinese herbs. They are not vitamins, they are medicine. People often do not realize how strong the herbs are to enhance healing.

Taking herbs three times a day is almost like getting acupuncture three times a day. Every time you take them, you are getting better, by addressing the root cause of the problem.

Licensed acupuncturists study Chinese herbal medicine for at least two years in acupuncture school. The first year is spent learning hundreds of individual herbs. Each herb has a function, temperature, organ affected, and how it is commonly used.

The chapter on how to find a great acupuncturist explains a lot more on acupuncture school training.

Stress Treatment Herbs

Stress can be relieved by taking Chinese herbs. The most common way the herbs are taken is in formulas. Each formula has four to 20 single herbs in it. Some formulas have dozens of single herbs. Each herb has a function in the formula. You can alter the effects of the herbal formula dramatically by adding a few additional herbs.

Chinese herbal medicine is available in patents and these are commonly purchased at Chinese grocery stores and pharmacies. The same way that you go to the store to buy aspirin for your headache, or drugs for you pain, traditionally Chinese people buy herbs for headaches, and herbs for pain. There are thousands of herbs available.

The most inexpensive type of herbal formula is called a "patent." That is also called a tea pill, or honey pill. Some companies use a lot of honey or other ingredients to make it less expensive. The word that tells you it is a teapill is "wan."

Chinese Patent Herbs

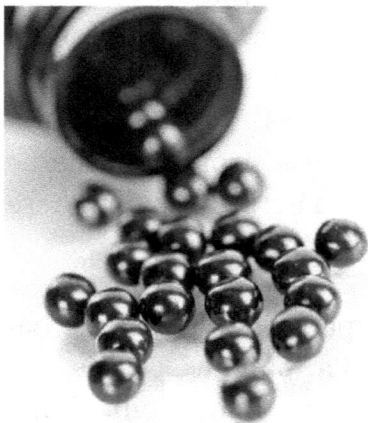

Acupuncturists can prescribe patent formulas from many different companies as appropriate. I sometimes prescribe pharmaceutical grade herbs such as Golden Flower Chinese Herbs, which is available only through licensed acupuncturists, and I might add a formula to address another health issue. So a patient might take a formula during the day that treats pain, but they can also take another formula with dinner and before bed for sleep. That is how I often treat multiple health issues at the same time. If you will be open to taking herbs, you will recover your health much faster.

Patent herbs have a wide range of prices. Each company has different formulas. A formula that includes Panax Ginseng, for example, will cost a little more than one that does not. I sometimes use formulas with no ginseng in them to treat patients with high blood pressure.

Please do not take Chinese Ginseng, also called Panax Ginseng, without a qualified herbalist prescribing it if you have high blood pressure. It makes your heart beat stronger, which can raise blood pressure in some people. Strengthening the heart muscle is great for health, but if you do that with someone who has high blood pressure, it can cause problems.

Chinese herbs for stress can vary a lot in ingredients. There is a basic formula called Xiao Yao Wan, or Free and Easy Wanderer. That is a very popular formula for over the counter usage. There are much stronger formulas that can be used for stress, but that formula is very balanced, which means it is less likely to cause side effects.

If you take the exact correct formula for your illness, you will recover faster. It is not uncommon to take a different herbal formula every week, and get acupuncture on different points also.

If you see several different acupuncturists, you will notice each acupuncturist will likely use different acupuncture points, and different herbs. That is because there are many ways to use acupuncture and no two treatments would be alike. That does not mean that one treatment was wrong, only that was what was chosen for that patient at that point in time. It is good to change things up and see if you can get a shift even better than the last one. There are over 400 points on the body. I have included the most common points in my point location book, *Acupuncture Points Handbook*.

However, if you include all the different types of acupuncture, there are actually thousands of acupuncture points on the body.

Chapter 9

Best Acupressure Points for Headaches

In order to get good results with acupressure, it is important to stimulate the points strongly enough to activate them. When acupuncture is done, the needle is inserted, adjusted a little, and then left in for 20 to 30 minutes to process. That gives the body enough time to process the treatment points.

There are over 100 points on the body that treat headaches. There are points that treat the head in general, and points that address different areas of the head. I am including in this chapter only the points that I believe can be treated effectively with acupressure.

Acupressure Point Stimulation Options

1. Press and massage the point for at least five minutes. You can alternate sides. Start with the left side and switch to the right side.
2. Use a mini massager. These massagers have interchangeable heads. I prefer the one with the most prongs on it for acupressure.

I have put links to massagers on my website, www.acupunctureexplained.com. It is not necessary to us a mini massager, but I have found the results are more dependable.

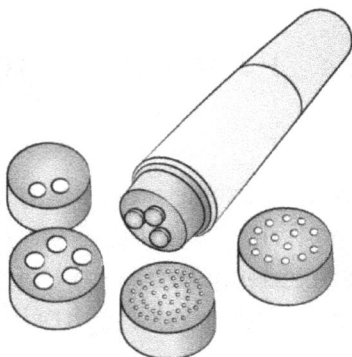

Large Intestine 4, Master Head Point

Large intestine 4 is located on the hand. You might have seen an image of this point in an article on acupressure. It is one of the most commonly known acupuncture points. It is called the "master point of the head." That means that it can be used for any problem on the head. It is sometimes used to perform dental surgery and other types of surgery.

Large Intestine 4

Allergies
Headaches
Colds and Flu
Face Point
Immune System

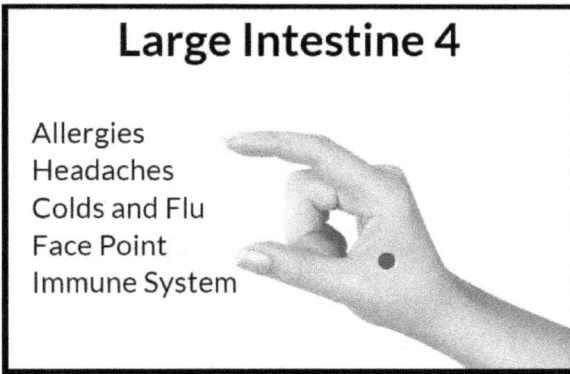

There are many commonly used points on the hands and feet. They are easy to access, and easy to treat with acupressure.

There are points between the toes for example that are too tight to use anything but a needle on. So try the acupressure points listed here, but your acupuncturist will be able to treat many more points.

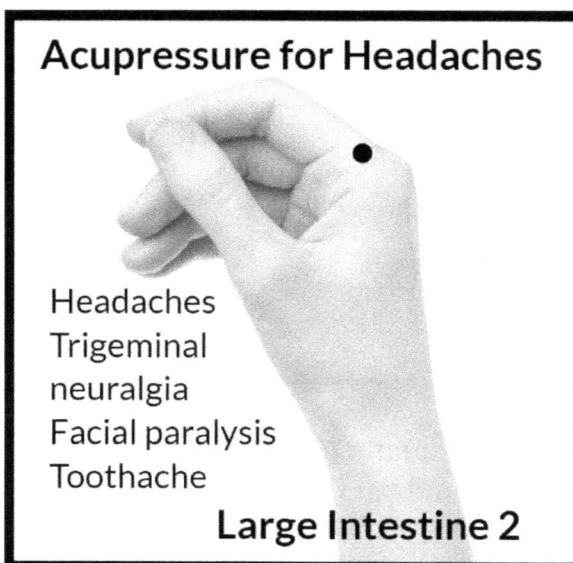

Acupressure for Headaches

Headaches
Trigeminal
neuralgia
Facial paralysis
Toothache

Large Intestine 2

Large intestine 2 is on the finger side of the knuckle, in other words just past the knuckle. It won't hurt if you treat a different point by mistake, but this is very effective for headaches.

The following points are from a special type of acupuncture, called Master Tung acupuncture. Master Tung was a famous acupuncturist in Taiwan. His family had been acupuncturists for over 2,000 years and they had their own system of acupuncture. They had developed acupuncture points that were kept as a family secret. This is not uncommon in China. Acupuncturists pass on family secrets for many generations. Fortunately for us, Master Tung shared his family secrets.

The following points are located on the fingers. Each finger is used to treat a headache on a specific part of the head, but considering most headaches originate from several locations, it is simpler to treat all the points. I believe a mini massager is the best way to treat these points. Press on each point for five minutes.

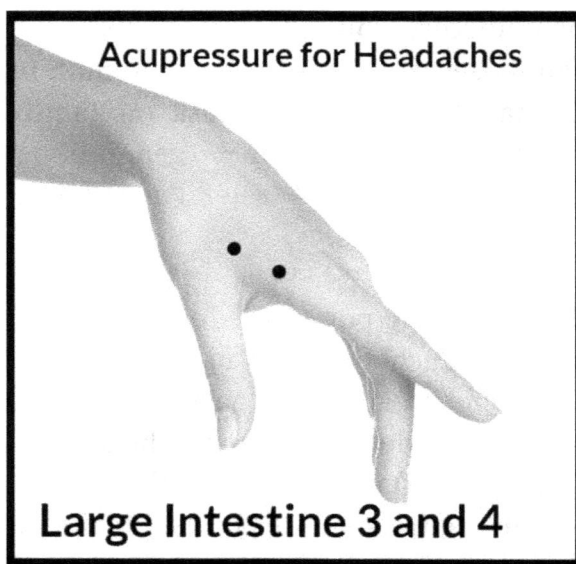

Acupressure for Headaches

Large Intestine 3 and 4

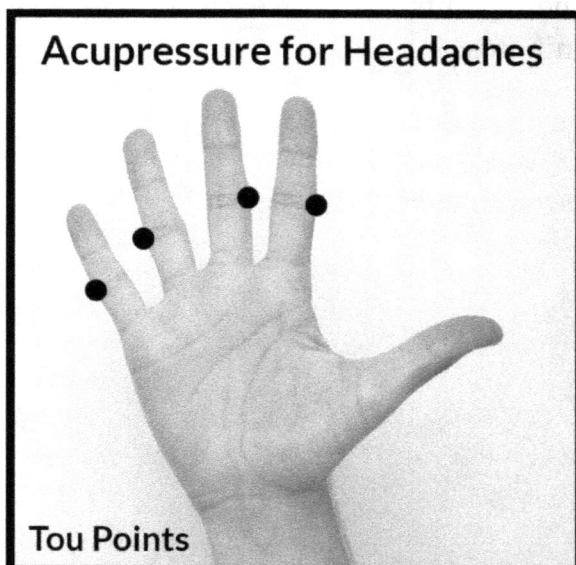

Acupressure for Headaches

Tou Points

These points are Tung acupuncture points. They are called Tou Points. That is pronounced "toe." I have several images of these points, to make it clear where they are located. Each point treats a different part of the head, but it is easy to just treat all of them, as it can be hard to determine which part of the head hurts worse, or where the pain originates.

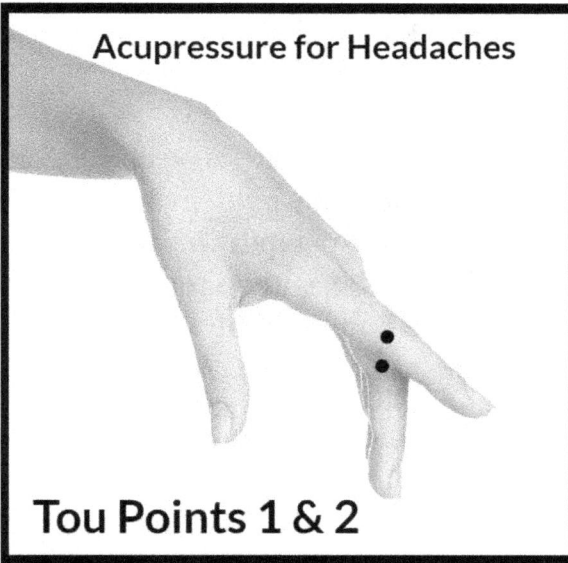

Acupressure for Headaches

Tou Points 1 & 2

Acupressure for Headaches

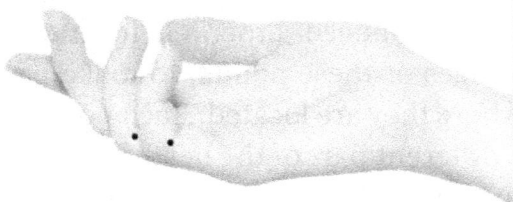

Tou Points 3 & 4

The first two points, one and two, are located on the thumb side of the knuckle. Points three and four are located on the little finger side.

The base of the head is where many muscles attach. I would include these points for most types of migraines. Lying down relaxes the muscles so you can feel them more easily. Be gentle in this area, as it is very sensitive. Just press on each point about five minutes.

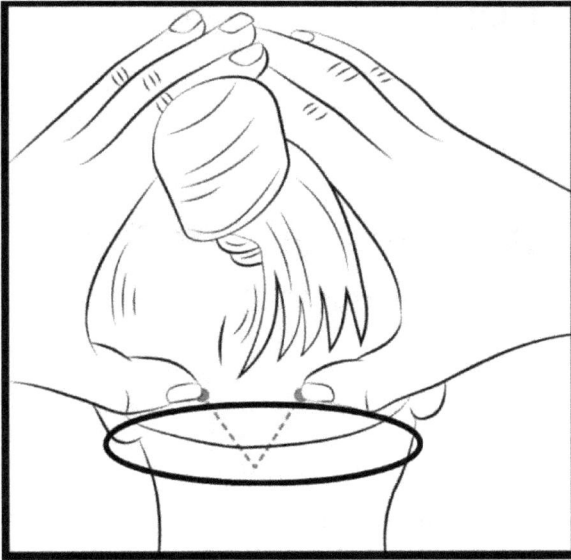

Please bear in mind that these acupressure points are meant to be used in addition to getting acupuncture. Your acupuncturist might have additional points to recommend, depending on which meridians are blocked in your case.

Chapter 10

Acupressure for Sinus Headaches

In addition to the regular points for headaches, there are several acupressure points that are effective for sinus problems.

The best points for sinus headaches are near or on the nose. A popular point is Large Intestine 20. It is located very close to the nose. This point usually works within a few minutes. You can feel your sinuses drain, unless you have a large amount of thick mucus in them. Herbal formulas will be prescribed that treat sinus inflammation for lasting relief.

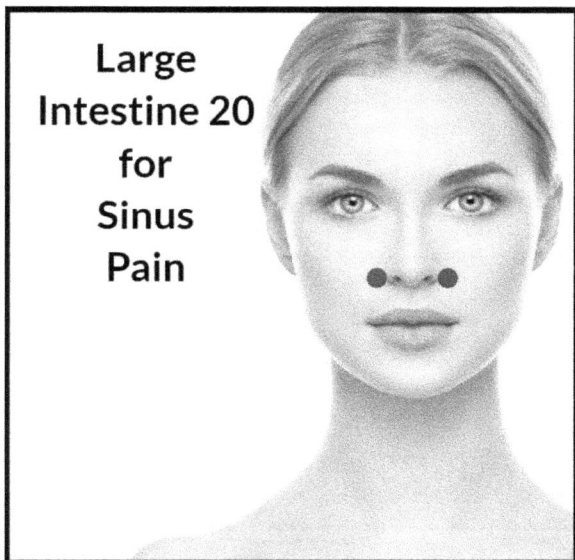

Large Intestine 20 for Sinus Pain

Additional points for sinus headaches are located on the nose and above it. Here is the sinus image again:

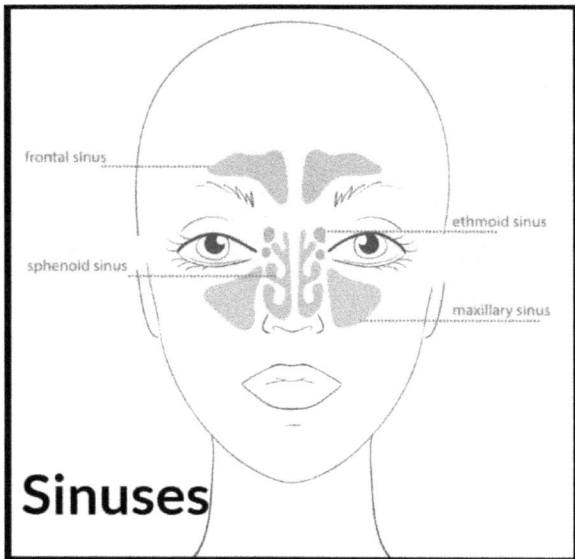

frontal sinus

ethmoid sinus

sphenoid sinus

maxillary sinus

Sinuses

If you notice, there are upper sinuses above the eyebrows. It is hard to tell exactly which sinuses are blocked, they might all be blocked. So it is best to treat all of them. The following points are extremely effective to relieve sinus pain.

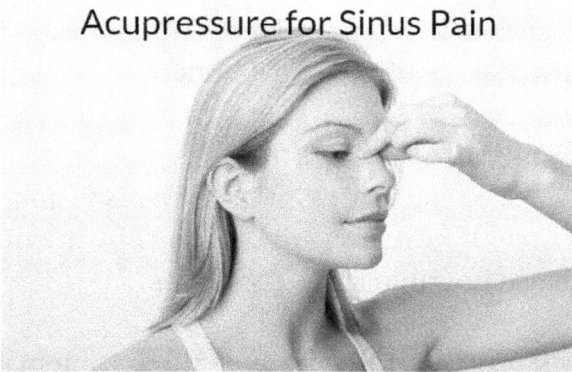

Acupressure for Sinus Pain

Here is another image of the points:

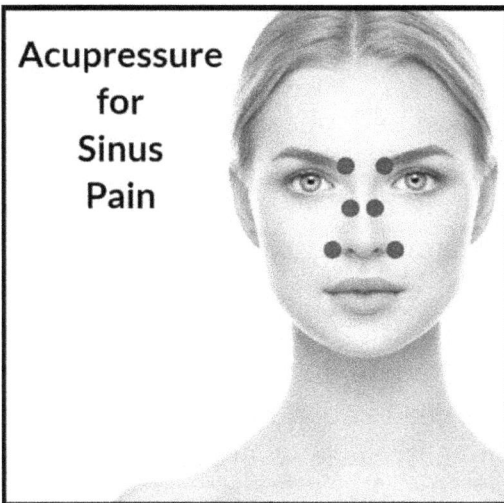

Acupressure for Sinus Pain

You can just squeeze the bridge of the nose as the model is showing. You will feel the sinus bone. The point is located at the edge of the sinus bone.

Dust Mite Allergens

Another cause for sinus problems is dust mites. If you are sensitive to this, it can cause horrible sinus problems.

My dad had horrible sinus problems with non-stop sneezing every day. When I visited him one time, I noticed that his sneezing was worse when he sat in the living room.

He had an old pheasant fabric couch with a hide a bed in it. When I slept on it I had sinus headaches and my sinuses actually completely closed up one day. I did some research and determined that old furniture can have a large accumulation of dust mite poo. The dust mites are bad enough, but their poo can build up and cause severe allergies.

Determining that the cause of his problem was the old pheasant couch he was so determined to keep was enough to convince him to get a new one.

If you have an old bed, or other fabric furniture, it might be making you sick. There are special bed bags and pillow bags that can be used that prevent the dust mites from getting through.

You can also buy natural dust mite killer. But you cannot get rid of them completely, they feed on your dead skin cells that flake off daily. I know that is gross, but they are cleaning your house every day. We used the Ecology works brand, but there are many to choose from. Dust mites are one of the most common allergens in the house.

I would vacuum as well as you can, using a HEPA filter vacuum cleaner, then apply dust mite killer as directed. After their numbers have been reduced, you can take action to get rid of the old furniture, or cover it with a sheet or couch cover if you cannot replace it.

Your bed is also a common problem area. If you are reacting to dust mites, I would consider encasing the mattress in a dust mite cover, and getting new pillows and pillow cases that block dust mites and other allergens.

Chapter 11

Acupressure for Food Allergies

As mentioned earlier, food allergies can easily cause sinus pain, as well as headaches. There are different therapies that treat all types of allergies, like NAET, which stands for Nambudripad Allergy Elimination Technique.

This treatment involves being tested to determine what the allergies are, and being treated by holding a vial that represents the allergen. The points along the spine are stimulated with a massager while you hold the vial. This actually "reboots" your body's reaction to the allergen. You then avoid the allergen for 25 hours after your treatment, and your body will not experience the same allergic reactions.

Although the process involves more points, I have found that there are two points that can be effective using acupressure. I do not suggest exposing yourself to the thing you are allergic to for this treatment, but simply massaging the points calms down the immune system. You can use your fingers, they points are very strong and they do not need a lot of stimulation to work.

The first point to use for allergies is Large Intestine 4. This point is one of the most famous acupuncture points. It is used to treat any problem on the head, allergies, sinus, hand pain, and many other things. My point location book lists dozens of actions of this point, but the ones relevant to this chapter are included on the image.

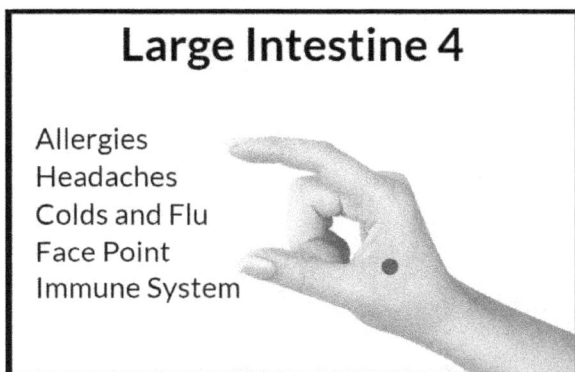

Large Intestine 4

Allergies
Headaches
Colds and Flu
Face Point
Immune System

I usually press firmly and rub the point for about five minutes on each side. This treats allergies and headaches at the same time. There is no harm in massaging the points for longer. Remember that acupuncture lasts about 30 minutes. The needles are inserted and left in for 30 minutes. For some conditions they are not left in that long, but that is the most common.

The other point that treats allergies is Large Intestine 11. This point is great for allergies, colds and flu, constipation, and fever.

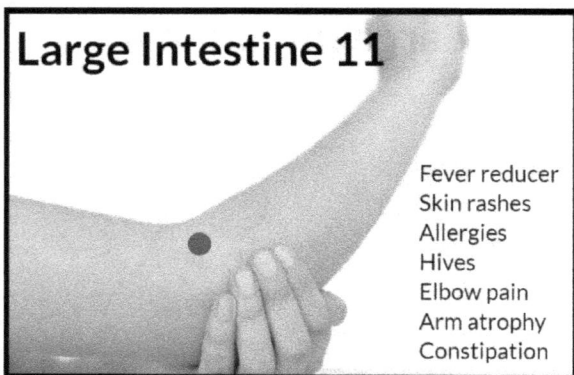

Large Intestine 11

Fever reducer
Skin rashes
Allergies
Hives
Elbow pain
Arm atrophy
Constipation

Food allergies are very serious. If you have a reaction to something, stop eating it immediately. Every time you eat it, your body can react more strongly. Leaky gut is often a factor in food allergies. The most important thing to consider for food allergies is taking high quality probiotics. I like the Garden of Life Primal Defense Ultra. This is the best product I have found to restore the intestines. There is a book about leaky gut called *Eat Dirt*, by Dr. Josh Axe. It explains leaky gut in detail.

Large Intestine 4 and 11 are helpful for allergies to cigarette smoke also. If you are exposed to smoke, you might get relief from the symptoms using acupressure until you can get away from it.

Cigarette and cigar smoke are toxic, so I doubt that you can stop reacting to it completely if you are exposed to it again, but you can treat yourself with acupuncture and get relief.

One of my patients takes the Jade Screen and Xanthium formula from Golden Flower Chinese Herbs when she has to go to an area where there will be cigarette smoke. She does not react to the smoke when she takes her herbs before she goes. This brand is only available through Licensed Acupuncturists. It treats allergies and sinus problems. Your acupuncturist might have an herbal formula she prefers for this problem.

Chapter 12

Acupressure for Seasonal Allergies

Seasonal or year round allergies can be treated with acupuncture and herbs. It is helpful to have a bottle of herbs handy to use if your allergies flare up. There are acupuncture points that boost your immune system and relieve the symptoms of allergies.

The strongest points for your immune system were mentioned in the sinus chapter, but I will add them here, Large Intestine 4 and 11.

The acupressure points in this book are only to tide you over while you get care from a licensed acupuncturist.

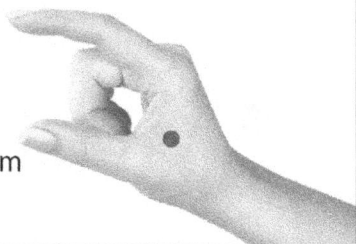

Large Intestine 4

Allergies
Headaches
Colds and Flu
Face Point
Immune System

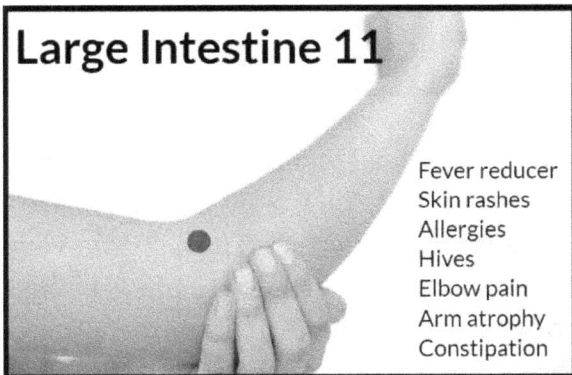

Large Intestine 11

Fever reducer
Skin rashes
Allergies
Hives
Elbow pain
Arm atrophy
Constipation

In addition to these points, there are points on the leg that are important.

The first point is Stomach 36. This is one of the most important points on the body. It boosts the immune system, improves digestion, treats fatigue, and regulates the intestines. There are dozens of functions of this point listed in *Acupuncture Points Handbook*.

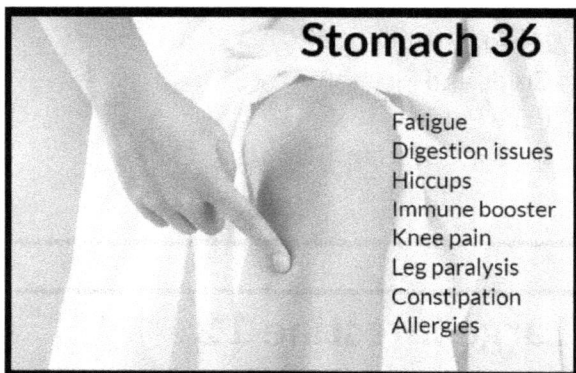

Stomach 36

Fatigue
Digestion issues
Hiccups
Immune booster
Knee pain
Leg paralysis
Constipation
Allergies

Stomach 36 is located just below the knee. You will feel a little hollow area there when you press. The point is very large, so it would be hard to miss it when you do acupressure. This point is used for most acupuncture treatments. My teacher, Dr. Wu, was quoted as saying that people need it "if they are human beings." It does more than could ever be listed in a book.

The other major point is called the "phlegm point." It is called that because it actually dissolves phlegm (mucus) in the lungs, and systemically. If you have a lot of mucus from allergies, a cold or flu, or some other issue, this point will help resolve it. After treating it people will often start coughing. That is the body trying to expel the mucus. It is located halfway along the calf.

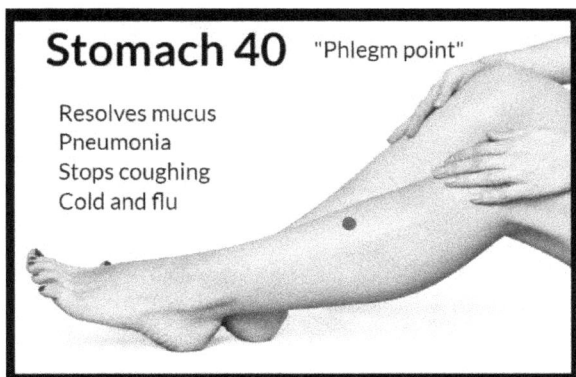

Stomach 40 "Phlegm point"

Resolves mucus
Pneumonia
Stops coughing
Cold and flu

I once treated a five year old boy who could not play outside. His mother was desperate to help him have a normal life. I prescribed a simple herbal formula called Jade Windscreen. This formula has immune tonic herbs like astragalus in it. Within a month he was able to play outside with no symptoms. He simply needed something to boost his immune system. Since he was so young, he responded quickly to a simple herbal formula. For adults I would usually have to use stronger formulas, because as we age our immune system tends to get weaker. Fortunately we have Chinese herbs to treat that.

Chapter 13

Acupressure for Neck Pain

If you have neck pain, a tight neck, or tight shoulders, this can easily cause headaches. In addition to the following acupressure points and getting acupuncture, there are other things that relieve neck pain.

Heat Wraps

One of my favorite remedies for neck pain is Thermacare heat wraps. They make a wrap for the neck, and one for the shoulders. When you open them they heat up. This might sound like it is too simple to help, but heat relaxes the muscles. Applying gentle heat for a few hours can relax tight muscles. When you heat an area, it improves blood flow. That enables the muscles to relax.

I have used this myself to treat sudden stiff neck. For other types of neck pain I like to use the ear seeds. That is very effective. In my office, I use far infrared heat lamps to treat most types of pain. It improves blood flow and relaxes the muscles. The benefit of using Thermacare patches is that you don't have to sit in one place, and they easily conform to your body.

When I have used these patches, I make sure the heat patch goes all the way to the base of the skull. That is where muscles attach, and I like to cover the whole area.

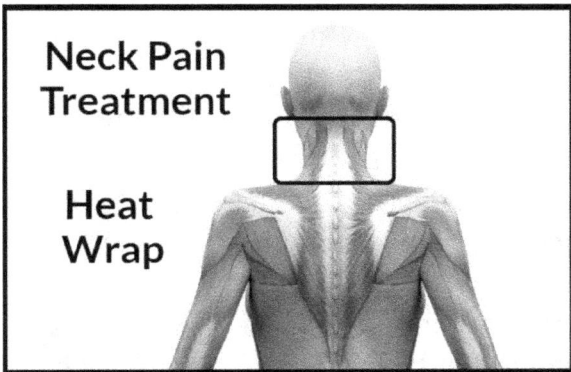

I believe many migraine sufferers could benefit from using gentle heat on the neck and shoulders.

There are numerous points on the body that treat neck pain. There are more options using acupuncture needles, but I wanted to include the points most likely to be effective with acupressure.

At the base of your head, at the hairline in the back, is where major muscles attach. Massaging this area gently, especially when lying down, is helpful to relax these muscles. When the muscles are tight in this area, it can cause dizziness, and ear problems.

The image below shows the acupuncture point Gallbladder 20, but I would massage all the points in that area. You will find sore spots. That tells you there is a problem in that area. I have found acupuncture in this location to be very effective for migraines. It relaxes the muscles and breaks down scar tissue, which can be created after muscles have been tight for a long time. I don't know if you could really call it scar tissue, but it is areas of very tight muscles, that feel like hard knots.

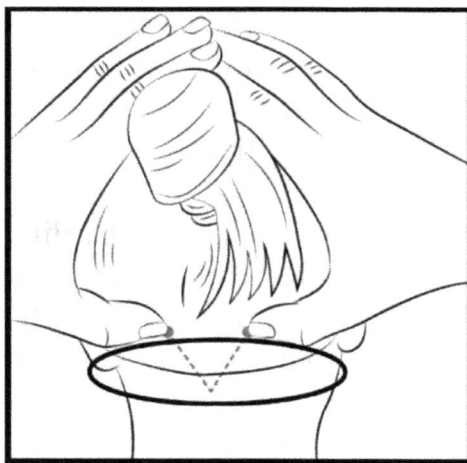

A common cause of headaches is when the atlas, or the area of cervical vertebrae 1 is too tight. If you have had a car accident or other injury, the joint can be slightly out of position, which causes pain.

I once had a chiropractor use an activator on the base of my skull. For three weeks I was dizzy. I finally had to do acupuncture in this area to relieve the pressure on the nerves, and the dizziness went away. It is easy to be too aggressive in this sensitive area of your body.

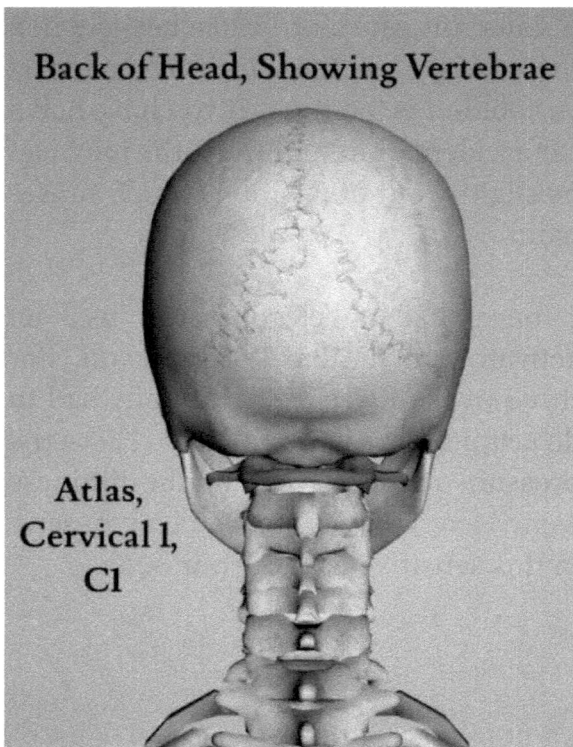

Back of Head, Showing Vertebrae

Atlas,
Cervical 1,
C1

The first area to treat with acupressure is the back of the head, where the muscles attach.

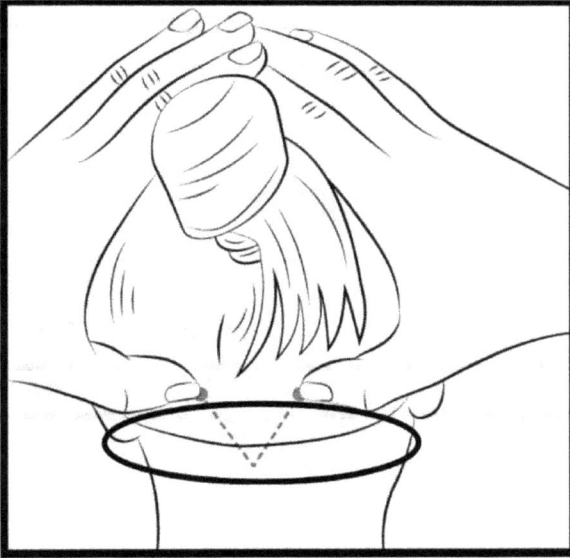

There are other points that are used to treat neck pain. I am not sure if acupressure will work on them, but I wanted to mention them. On the side of the hand, by the little finger, there are several points that are used to treat the neck. I believe you could use a mini massager on these points.

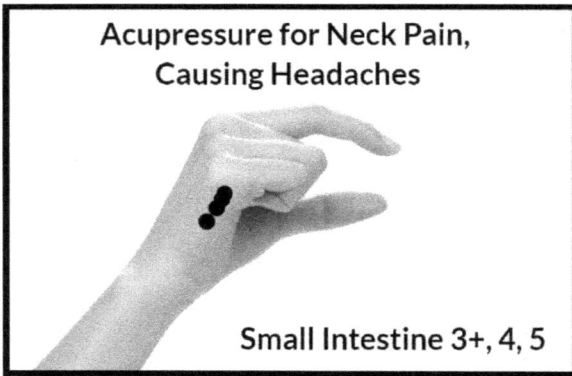

Acupressure for Neck Pain, Causing Headaches

Small Intestine 3+, 4, 5

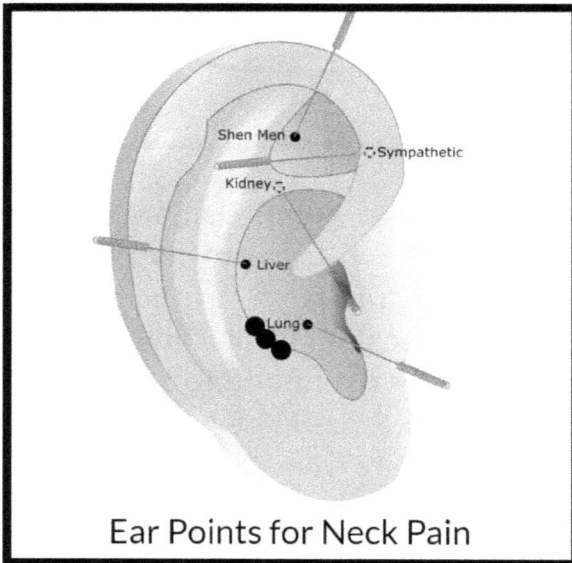

Ear Points for Neck Pain

This image shows where the neck can be treated on the ear.

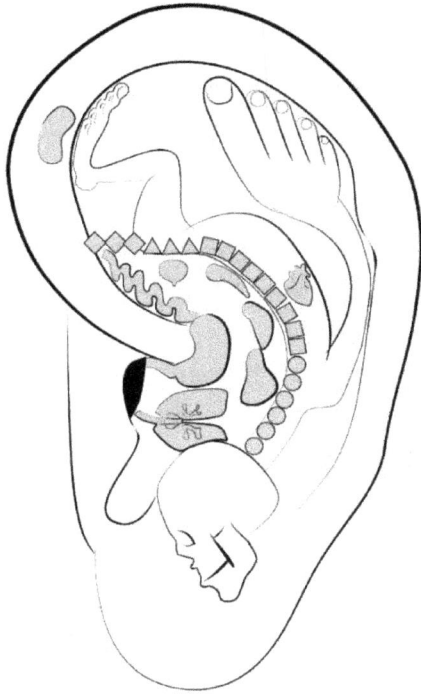

This image of the ear shows the upside down, or inverted fetus. There are acupuncturists who only use the ear to treat all ailments. Some acupuncturists like to add ear points as needed. I like to use little gold pellets to treat neck pain. Anything you can do to relax the neck and treat neck pain will help relieve migraines.

I place the gold or silver pellets on one ear, and then alternate ears for each treatment. Patients can press on the seeds to treat their own neck pain.

You can use other types of pellets. Traditionally ear seeds are placed on a piece of tape. Vaccaria seeds are used. The seeds continue to put gentle pressure on the ear to treat the problem, even if you do not press on it, but you will usually notice a bigger difference if you press on it.

I use Sakamura ionic ear seeds. They come with either flesh colored tape, or clear tape. Ear acupuncture is a way to treat yourself at home. However the ear is very small and it is not always easy to find the points if you are not trained for that. Treating the neck and back via the ear is pretty easy. The spine is represented on the ridge of the ear, and it is easy to locate.

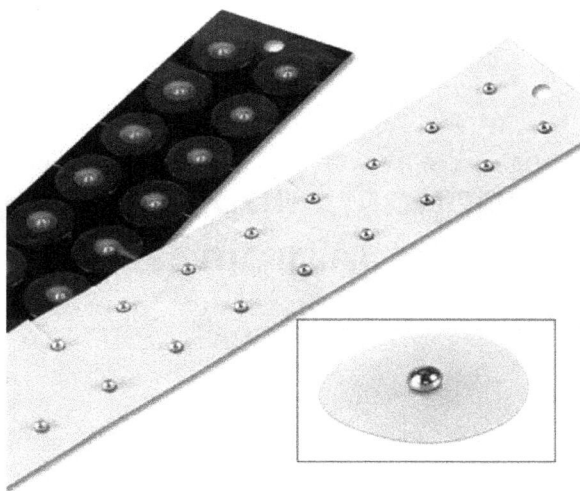

Sakamura ear pellets

Chapter 14

Important Supplements for Migraines

The most important supplement for migraine patients to take is magnesium. Your muscles cannot relax without magnesium. About 80% of Americans do not have enough magnesium. This causes many health problems.

Some people take calcium supplements that do not contain magnesium. This is a bad idea. Calcium needs magnesium and other cofactors like Vitamin D to be absorbed.

A common cause of calcium and magnesium deficiency is drinking soft drinks. They contain phosphoric acid, which has to be buffered by calcium. If you do not take enough, your body pulls the minerals from your bones. If you have ever consumed soft drinks regularly, it would be a good idea to take a good supplement for a while.

Raw Calcium

My favorite calcium and magnesium supplement is Raw Calcium from Garden of life. It is organic, and contains all the necessary cofactors for absorption. The dosage is 4 capsules per day.

I had a patient who had hip pain that would go away for a while, then come back later. This did not make sense. Normally the pain goes away and does not come back after a course of treatment. We determined that she had osteoporosis and the bone in her hip was dissolving, which was irritating the tissue. Once she took a good quality calcium and magnesium supplement for a while, the pain finally went away completely. Osteoporosis can cause tiny bone fragments to inflame local tissue.

This can cause pain anywhere in the body.

Magnesium oxide is commonly used in supplements. It is not well absorbed. If you find a supplement with magnesium oxide on the ingredient list, I would steer clear of that.

Chelated Magnesium Glycinate

Chelated magnesium glycinate is the best absorbed magnesium. I like the Doctor's Best brand. It is inexpensive, and very effective. If you read the testimonials, you will see some people cured their migraines by taking this type of magnesium. Be sure to take the full dosage of this supplement. You might consider taking a couple tablets in the morning, and a couple in the evening.

Magnesium Malate

Another type of magnesium that works well is magnesium malate. This type has been used for years by fibromyalgia sufferers. It is especially good to relax the muscles and some people find that it helps them relax well enough to sleep.

The importance of taking magnesium cannot be overstated. Even if you hate taking pills, most people should take it at least a month to ensure adequate supply. Nurses often test for magnesium levels when you go to the hospital. They supply magnesium by IV to treat some diseases.

I usually recommend Raw Calcium for all my female patients. I would then add the magnesium glycinate, especially in the evening.

The only way you will know if you are magnesium deficient and that is causing your migraines, is if you take the supplements and find out. I would err on the side of taking them to see if they will help.

If you prefer to take a liquid supplement, Natural Calm is a powder that you can mix yourself. It is made by Natural Vitality.

If you are on any medications, of course consult your doctor on supplements.

Sinus Supplements

If you have sinus issues, you can get herbal formulas from your licensed acupuncturist. There are also formulas that are sold over the counter. I believe they are not as effective as the brands your acupuncturist can buy, but they are something to consider. Butterbur has been used for years to treat migraines.

Garden of Life makes a product called Natural Sinus Support. This product includes enzymes that relieve inflammation. It also contains butterbur extract, vitamin C, and probiotics.

There is a theory in Western medicine that the cause of migraines is inflamed veins. They don't correlate this to the root cause of the inflammation, which is tight muscles and lack of healthy blood flow.

Ginger Root Extract

Anti-inflammatory herbs like ginger root can be very effective pain relievers. You can buy ginger root that is the raw herb chopped up and encapsulated. This product is available at most stores. I have not taken the brands sold at discount stores or drugstores, but I suspect they should be OK. It is hard to mess up ginger root.

A better option is to take ginger root extract. That is made by boiling ginger root and taking the liquid from that and making it into capsules and tablets. Extracts are four to five times as strong as the raw herb products. This means that you won't have to take as many pills. Instead of 4 capsules of ginger root, you can take one ginger root extract pill.

Jarrow and Planetary Herbals make great ginger root extract products. Jarrow ginger is in capsules. Their concentrate is 4 to 1. That means that each capsule is about the same as 4 capsules of the raw root.

The Planetary Herbals product is in tablet form. When I take ginger extract I take 2-3 tablets at a time. It is also the number one remedy for diarrhea. If you catch colds and flus and allergies early, ginger root might knock it out. It also boosts stomach acid secretion, so it improves digestion. Ginger should be taken with food in most cases.

Bupleurum Calmative
There are Chinese herbs that relieve stress, by regulating the liver energy. Planetary Herbals makes several great herbal formulas. The one that correlates to Xiao Yao San is called Bupleurum Calmative.

Your acupuncturist will prescribe formulas that more precisely match your problems, but if you do not have access to an acupuncturist immediately, I wanted to give you information on a quality product.

This is what Planetary Herbals says about their formula:

"Planetary Herbals **Bupleurum Calmative Compound** is based on a classic Chinese herbal preparation (*Xiao Yao Wan*) which has been known under various names, such as "Relaxed Wanderer" and "Free and Relaxed Pills." It was developed in the Song Dynasty (960-1279) almost 875 years ago. Especially useful for premenstrual and menopausal ups and downs, it has remained one of Chinese herbalism's most valued formulas for supporting a calm state of emotional well-being."

Notice that this formula was developed around 875 years ago!

This formula can increase fertility, so take precautions if you do not want to get pregnant.

The following are the ingredients:

Proprietary Blend: Dong Quai Root, Bai-Zhu Atractylodes Rhizome, Chinese Peony Root, Poria Sclerotium, Ginger Root Extract, Licorice Root Extract,

Chinese Mint Aerial Parts, and Bupleurum Root Extract.

This formula should not be combined with any drugs, or used by pregnant or nursing women. This is for informational purposes only.

Chapter 15

How to Find a Great Acupuncturist and How Much Acupuncture Costs

When you look for a great acupuncturist, you will want to ask what type of license and education the person has. Most states in America call acupuncturists Licensed Acupuncturists. The state ensures they have a three to four year Master's Degree in Oriental Medicine, and that they pass national tests that show competency in Chinese medicine.

In acupuncture school we spend the first year learning:

- 400 acupuncture points
- How to locate acupuncture points
- What angle the needle is inserted for safety
- How deep the needle goes in for over 400 points
- What functions each point has
- How to combine acupuncture points for the best results
- How to diagnose disease using Chinese medicine principles

The second year:

- How to treat many diseases
- Single Chinese herbs, what each herb does
- Start student clinic treating patients under the supervision of an experienced acupuncturist

The third year:

- Herbal formulas are learned. We learn how each herb is combined into formulas to treat disease
- Student clinic full time

- Treating disease with Chinese medicine

This is a very basic breakdown. Our classes also include Western Medicine, anatomy and physiology, and many other topics. The point is that this is a complicated and wonderful medicine.

The people who have a Master Degree in Oriental Medicine are very qualified to help you. When you call a person who does acupuncture, ask her if she is licensed to do acupuncture, and if she has a degree in Chinese medicine. This is not the same thing as a "certification," which often entails taking a few weekend classes in acupuncture.

I once observed a chiropractor insert needles into a person's shoulder in such a way that I doubted there would be any benefit. The angle of insertion was also unusual. She inserted needles into the shoulder at the wrong angle, which could have pierced the upper lobe of the lung. She did not have proper acupuncture training, as it was not required by the state she practiced in at the time.

In acupuncture school we learn how to insert the needles safely and correctly. I personally believe that other healthcare providers should pass a state supervised training. They should take a minimum of two years of acupuncture school. They can skip the Western medicine and anatomy classes, but the training should be standardized, and they should be tested. There are people prescribing Chinese herbs who do not know what they are doing. Licensed acupuncturists study herbs for two solid years in school.

1. Ask if the person has a state license in acupuncture
2. Ask if the person has a degree in Chinese medicine

That is what you need to know about the process of finding a great acupuncturist.

To find a great acupuncturist, you want to look for the initials LAc. This means Licensed Acupuncturist. Acupuncture school is a graduate level program that lasts at least three years. Other types of practitioners do acupuncture, but did they attend school for three years? That is the most important thing to ask. Ask the person if they went to acupuncture school and have a degree in Chinese medicine.

Each state has a different designation for acupuncturists. In Rhode Island, acupuncturists are called Doctors of Acupuncture. In New Mexico, acupuncturists are considered primary care doctors and are called Doctors of Oriental Medicine, or DOM. Most states call acupuncturists LAc, or Licensed Acupuncturists.

If someone says he is "certified" in acupuncture, ask what that means. There are weekend classes that "certify" chiropractors and other healthcare providers to do acupuncture. This does not mean they attended acupuncture school with thousands of hours of training.

ACUPUNCTURE FOR MIGRAINES

I wanted to include the curriculum for the AOMA acupuncture school. This is an example how what Licensed Acupuncturists study for three to four years. I copied this directly from their website at www.aoma.edu. This is the school I attended, and I highly recommend it.

<u>Acupuncture Studies and Chinese Medicine Fundamentals</u>

The foundations and diagnostic skills of traditional Chinese medicine are the fundamental cornerstone of Chinese medical science. This theoretical system forms the basis for clinical practice. The well-rounded and comprehensive acupuncture curriculum builds on these fundamentals, creating a strong foundation for other didactic instruction and for clinical internship.

- Introduction to Palpation
- Foundations of Chinese Medicine 1
- Foundations of Chinese Medicine 2

140

- Diagnostic Skills of Chinese Medicine 1
- Diagnostic Skills of Chinese Medicine 2
- Point Location and Meridian Theory 1
- Point Location and Meridian Theory 2
- Point Location and Meridian Theory 3
- Acupuncture Techniques 1
- Acupuncture Techniques 2
- Meridian and Point Energetics 1
- Meridian and Point Energetics 2
- Advanced Needling Techniques and Theory
- Acupuncture Treatment of Disease 1
- Acupuncture Treatment of Disease 2
- Acupuncture Treatment of Disease 3
- NCCAOM Board Exams Preparation
- Additional Acupuncture Courses available as electives

Herbal Studies

AOMA's herbal program is one of the most comprehensive in the nation, with education in the theory, identification, and

141

function of more than 300 herbs and the combination of those herbs in formulas to restore states of health. Resources include an herbal lab, an herbal medicine center which stocks more than 350 herbs in bulk and powdered form, patent formulas, tablets, capsules, and extracts, and a learning garden where herbs are grown in conjunction with the American Botanical Council.

- Chinese Herbology 1
- Chinese Herbal Studies Lab 1
- Nutrition and Dietary Therapy
- Chinese Herbology 2
- Chinese Herbal Studies Lab 2
- Chinese Herbology 3
- Chinese Herbal Studies Lab 3
- Chinese Herbal Formulations 1
- Chinese Patent Herbal Medicine
- Chinese Herbal Formulations 2
- Chinese Herbal Formulations 3
- Syndrome-based Herbs and Formulas
- Chinese Herbal Safety & Herb-Drug Interactions
- Chinese Herbal Treatment of Disease 1
- Chinese Herbal Treatment of Disease 2

- Huang Di Nei Jing
- Shan Han Lun
- Chinese Herbal Treatment of Disease 3
- Jin Gui Yao Lue
- Wen Bing and Wen Re

Biomedical Sciences

AOMA's biomedical sciences curriculum provides students with a practical foundation of the concepts and diagnostic techniques of biomedicine, enabling them to interface successfully with allopathic practitioners. It is intended to provide students with information applicable to their Chinese medical practice upon becoming licensed practitioners and to enhance their ability to communicate with patients and other practitioners regarding biomedical diagnoses and treatment plans.

- Anatomy, Physiology and Histology 1
- Anatomy Lab 1
- Anatomy and Physiology 2
- Anatomy Lab 2
- Anatomy and Physiology 3

- Medical Biology
- Medical Biochemistry
- Biomedical Terminology
- Public Health and Biomedical Survey
- Microbiology and General Pathophysiology
- Systemic Pathophysiology
- Biomedical Pharmacology
- Biomedical Diagnostic Techniques: Body Imaging, Fluids Analysis and Lab Reports
- Physical Assessment 1
- Physical Assessment 2
- Evidence-Based Medicine in CAM Practice
- Women's Health: Management of Gynecological and Reproductive Conditions
- Biomedical Treatment of Disease, Segment 1
- Biomedical Treatment of Disease, Segment 2

MAcOM Graduation Requirements

The Master of Acupuncture and Oriental Medicine program must be completed within eight calendar years from the date of enrollment and within six years for students on federal financial aid. The following requirements must be met in order to graduate from the program:

Completion of all didactic and clinical instruction listed below:

	Credits	Hours
Acupuncture	63.5	768
Herbal	45	558
Integral	11	132
Biomedicine	42	504
Clinical	42	1008
Total	203.5	2970

Licensed Acupuncturist (LAc)

- Average of 2,700+ hours of master's level training
- Master's level, on-site training at a nationally accredited school or college of acupuncture
- Hundreds of hours of clinical experience and at least 250 actual patient treatments before licensure
- Required to pass the national certification exam in acupuncture in order to become licensed (NCCAOM)
- Required to do regular continuing education to maintain national certification

How Much Acupuncture Costs

Acupuncture ranges from $60 to $100 per visit. The cost of local rent and other expenses will be the biggest determining factor in many cases. Considering that you are getting treatment that will most likely cure your migraines for good, I think it is a bargain.

Here is how it works. Expect to get acupuncture at least twice a week for a month. For migraines, I would expect that you would need at least another four weeks. So budget for 16 visits. Let's say your acupuncturist charges $80 a visit. That is $1,280 for two months of care. You will usually pay separately for Chinese herbs. Each bottle is $15 or $20, and each bottle lasts about a week. So for less than $2,000, you should be able to be migraine free.

The maximum amount of time it usually takes for lasting relief is three months. You might be able to pre-pay for care and get a discount. If an acupuncturist knows you will stick to the treatment plan, get the acupuncture and herbs you need, they might offer a discount for paying up front. Doing this saves time and money for everyone. You do not have to pay each time you go in, so that can save 5-10 minutes per day. Your acupuncturist also might need to special order an herbal formula for you, so paying in advance makes it less likely that the special purchase is left on the shelf.

You will feel better soon after starting care, but to be migraine free will take two to three months of care.

That is two months of getting acupuncture for everything that is wrong with you. While getting migraine treatments, your stress is treated, sleep improves, hormones improve, and most ailments can be treated at the same time, depending on how bad it is. You might get acupuncture for your migraines, and take Chinese herbs to treat your insomnia or fatigue. It is truly a holistic treatment.

I had one patient who came to me after having a severe reaction to migraine drugs she was taking. She had to be rushed to the emergency room, she was throwing up and lost control of her bowels. Her part of the emergency room visit was $10,000. I believe that was for one day in the emergency room. I wish she had known about acupuncture a long time before she had that reaction and spent $10,000 on treatment that did not cure her. We were able to completely resolve her migraines in about two months. That means she no longer has to take any drugs, or see doctors, or take the chance she will react to pain drugs.

One of my migraine patients got pregnant after three months of acupuncture and herbs. She had been told she was infertile and could never get pregnant. She never expected to get pregnant.

If you do not want to get pregnant, be sure to use birth control when you get acupuncture. It strongly improves fertility, even when you are not trying to get pregnant. We cannot stop the improvement in fertility, because it is a natural side effect of acupuncture.

References

The *Foundations of Chinese Medicine*, by Giovanni Maciocia

Diagnosis in Chinese Medicine, by Giovanni Maciocia

The Practice of Chinese Medicine: The Treatment of Diseases with Acupuncture and Chinese Herbs, by Giovanni Maciocia

Giovanni Maciocia is the author of the majority of books used by acupuncturists to learn Chinese medicine. I recommend all his books. If you would like to learn Chinese medicine, the *Foundations of Chinese Medicine* book is the first year text. That is a good start.

ACUPUNCTURE
POINTS
HANDBOOK

A Patient's Guide
to the Locations and
Functions of Over
400
Acupuncture Points

DEBORAH BLEECKER, LAC, MSOM

Acupuncture Points Handbook is written for the non-acupuncturist. It explains each acupuncture point in an easy to understand way. If you ever wanted to know how each point works, this book will make it simple.

151

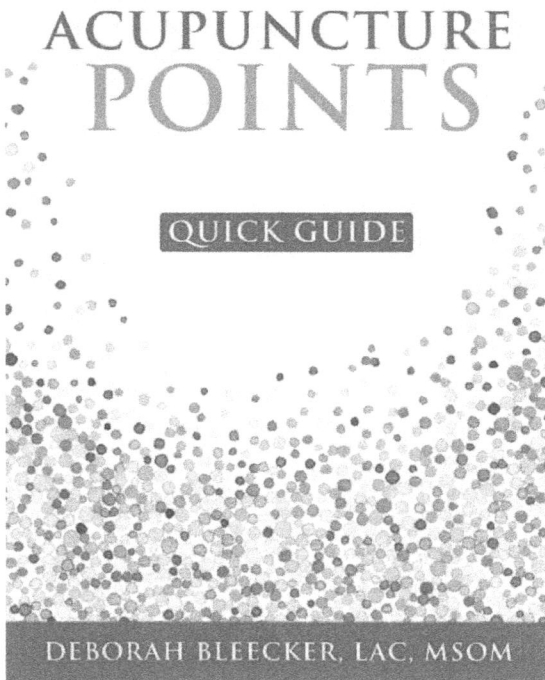

ACUPUNCTURE
POINTS

QUICK GUIDE

DEBORAH BLEECKER, LAC, MSOM

This book includes only the most important acupuncture points. Choose this if you want a quick guide to the most important points.

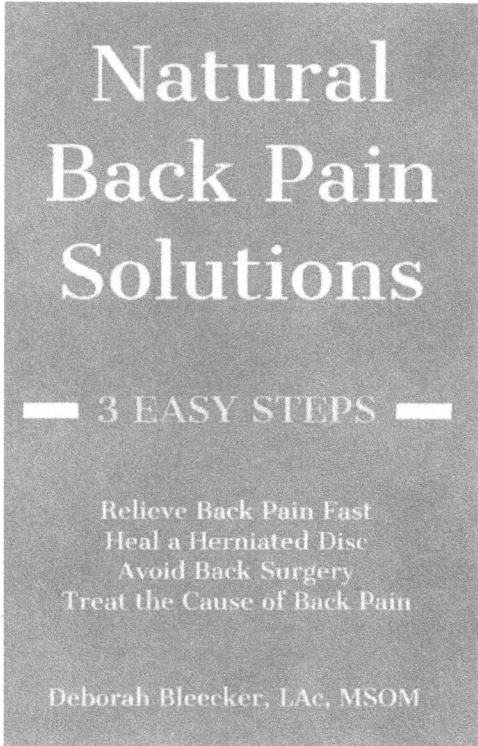

Natural Back Pain Solutions

▬ 3 EASY STEPS ▬

Relieve Back Pain Fast
Heal a Herniated Disc
Avoid Back Surgery
Treat the Cause of Back Pain

Deborah Bleecker, LAc, MSOM

This book includes everything you need to know about treating back pain effectively with natural remedies. Over one million people a year get surgery. Most of it is not necessary, and it causes permanent damage to tissue. Look for an alternative.

Shingles Relief

How to Relieve the Pain of Herpes Zoster, Treat the Herpes Virus, and Prevent Future Outbreaks

Deborah Bleecker, LAc, MSOM

Shingles is one of the worst diseases I have ever treated. There are natural treatment options, and ways to make a future outbreak less likely.

Index

155

Keep in Touch

I hope that you have benefitted from this book. My hope is that many people find this book and get out of pain fast. You can contact me at deborahbleecker@gmail.com.

You can find me at my main website, www.acupunctureexplained.com. I have placed videos and other content about this disease and others. You can also get a free e-book of the top five points in acupuncture, if you sign up for my mailing list.

Please consider leaving a review on Amazon for this book. I would appreciate the feedback. Thank you.

Acupuncture
Restores Healthy
Blood Flow to
Relieve Pain

Pain is Caused by a
Lack of Healthy
Blood Flow

www.ingramcontent.com/pod-product-compliance
Lightning Source LLC
Chambersburg PA
CBHW050127280326
41933CB00010B/1282